MEDICINE GROVE

MEDICINE GROVE

A Shamanic Herbal

Loren Cruden

Destiny Books
Rochester, Vermont

Destiny Books
One Park Street
Rochester, Vermont 05767
www.InnerTraditions.com

Destiny Books is a division of Inner Traditions International

LIBRARY OF CONGRESS CATALOGING-IN-PUBLICATION DATA

Cruden, Loren, 1952–
        Medicine grove : a shamanic herbal / Loren Cruden.
            p.   cm.
        Includes bibliographical references and index.
        ISBN 978-0-89281-647-7 (alk. paper)
        1. Herbs—Therapeutic use. 2. Shamanism. I. Title.
RM666.H33C78 1997   97-18606
615'.321—dc21   CIP

Printed and bound in the United States

10 9 8 7 6 5 4

Text design and layout by Kristin Camp
Photographs by Gabriel Cruden
This book was typeset in Palatino with Papyrus and Paleface as
    display faces

Table of Contents

Acknowledgments

The beautiful photographs are the work of my son, Gabriel Cruden. I am grateful for the way he sees, and shares his vision.

Gratitude to herbalists Susun Weed, Juliette de Bairacli Levy, Jeannine Parvati Baker, and the late David Forelines for renewing, extending, and sharing the spirit of alliance with plants.

Gratitude to those who have supported me through many years of difficulty and empty pockets, embodying the loving generosity that keeps life's web ashine: Robin, Axis, Jim and Tames, Susan, Joan, Denise, Stephanie and David, Liz, Catherine and Lawrence, Daryl, VJ, my beloved Vlodya, my son, and my parents, brothers, and sister.

Gratitude to the gracious trees and herbs, and to the mystery that dreams life.

Introduction

Direct acquaintance is the way to truly know plants. Shamanic relationship with plants emphasizes this: It is a relationship based on experiential and visionary knowledge. The shamanic way of working with herbs is an expression of cooperative healing; a way of partnership with the rooted beings that so gracefully sustain our earthly life.

Alliance with plants is an ancient art and survival skill. A great deal can be learned from studying how our ancestors, and the native peoples of North America, related to herbs and trees. Attending to that traditional knowledge is one facet of shamanic practice, but it is only through personal interaction with plants that authentic alliance can be cultivated; within that personal context comes the necessary teachings for efficacious practice. Through inquiring engagement the healer develops an understanding of and respect for individual plants based on truths of experience.

There are two primary schools of herbal practice: the naturalist school, which includes classical herbalism, ethnobotany, and the "wise woman" tradition; and the naturopathic school, which is the basis for most modern texts on herbology and for licensed herbal despensation in the United States. The naturopathic school also encompasses Christian herbalism, a kind of religious naturopathy, and what may be called "commercial" herbalism.

The naturalist school orients to health as an intrinsic though ever-varying state supported by integrated wholesome inter-action with habitat—herbs being a valued component of habitat. Emphasis is on tonics, nutrient plants, and botanicals that aid and nourish vital function. On the other hand, the naturo-pathic school, despite efforts at being holistic, views the body as a besieged temple with the colon as its desecrated sanctum. Emphasis is on purging toxins and cleansing the blood, lymph, and bowel—in short, the emphasis is on rectification.

Shamanic herbalism invites a third perspective, one con-cerned with healing relationship as a basis for health. This con-joins with the naturalist orientation but goes a step beyond, seeing herbs not only as an aspect of habitat but as a sentient tribe of beings.

Malidoma Patrice Somé, an African shaman, writes in his book *Of Water and the Spirit:*

> I remember the blind healer in the village who worked at night and slept during the day. The man was so skilled at conversing with trees that he baffled even his fellow medicine men with his spectacular talent for obtaining medicine from nature. His consultations always ended in the middle of the night. Then the patient was ordered to follow him into the bush. There he would speak to Mother Nature in a strange language, giving her a list of illnesses. She would respond in a buzzing language, telling him which plants he needed to gather.
>
> Then the vegetal world would awake in the middle of darkness, every tree and every plant—all speaking to the man at once. For the witness it was gibberish, but for the blind healer it made sense. He would translate, telling each patient that such and such a tree said his fruit dried and pounded and then mixed with salted water and drunk would take care of the disease in ques-tion. Another plant would say that it couldn't do any-thing by itself, but that if the patient could talk to an-other plant (whose name the healer knew) and mix their

substances together, their combined energies could kill such and such an illness.

Some trees said they were going through Amanda, a metamorphosis process that requires total seclusion. In such a state their vegetal substances could be very harmful. Yet other plants were busy helping their neighbors and could not help because of that. Their medicine, which did much good to the other trees, would be harmful to humans.

The healer was totally dependent on this dialogue with the vegetal in his work. He often said that the vegetal world was better than the human one because it knew more than we did, and because it is a finer species than we are. The vegetal can get along without us, but we cannot progress without the help of the vegetal.

The blind healer speaks of disease and cures, but what is foundational in this form of herbalism is knowledge of right relationship between species, within species, within tribe and self, and with Life as expressed through the cosmos.

Shamanic healing is directed toward the essential core of relationship, a causative level where patterns that define and interpret experience are formed from thought and belief. But the practice of shamanic healing in modern society exposes a dilemma. Modern consciousness habitually engages with a peripheral zone of complexity: symptoms, convoluted psychological constructs, material manifestations, reflexive emotional patterns, and so on. The drama of such complexity has a tremendous hold on modern minds. A person with an illness usually wants an apparent cure for an apparent condition, even though such a "cure" is almost always rather a temporary suppression of illness. Or those who are ill may be interested in discussing psychological implications of illness as ways of analyzing personality, identifying self through their disease or making it an absorbing nucleus around which orbit special diets, treatments, considerations, interactions with practitioners, and so on.

Healing on the causative or primal level necessitates changing the patterns that govern experience, and while most people in pursuit of healing claim to be seeking a state of complete wellness, this depth of healing is typically shied away from. Readiness to participate in actual change is rarely enough encountered that most practitioners and clients settle for gratifying, though temporary, fixes in peripheral zones, even when practitioners have skills and orientation that enable them to do core work with others.

Oftentimes treatment, whether with massage, herbs, or other physical modalities, catalyzes the surfacing and release of pent-up energies. These releases often accompanied by emotional catharsis can be useful, but they are mostly indicators of something deeper needing to be addressed, not transformative healings. They are like sand that has been piled on top of the body, bringing a tremendous weight and lack of mobility. When flung aside in the course of unburying, the sand's sudden removal brings relief, a lifting of pressure. But the sand is not the thing buried, and in a short while will start sliding back into the hole, covering again what lies inside.

Shamanic practice is hampered by a person's resistance to disengaging with complexity's drama, by fear of change, and by the cultural absence of models of right relationship ("right" not in a moralistic sense but in terms of Beauty, or essential harmony). In modern life, relationship is conceived of and internalized in dualistic terms: self or other, good or evil, healthy or sick, and so on. This orientation is the basis of modern religion and psychology, and thus is the paradigm carried over into most philosophies of healing, including alternative spirituality. Within that orientation, relationship is conceived of as a means for contrasting and comparing, or as a way of defining roles. Used this way, relationship distances through division or difference. For example, a person with manifestations of cancer is contrasted with a person not manifesting cancer, and relationship to health is measured on that basis. The contrast may also predicate relationship to self or to society.

When relationship is used to delineate roles or describe stasis, as in "our marriage relationship," the relationship becomes a thing possessed instead of an interaction; it becomes inert, an object instead of an activity. Dualism insists on distance, on egoic territorialism and fixed categorizations. It interprets relationship as something you personally have or don't have, or as a measure of difference, not as a universal dance in which you play a part. Relationship in the shamanic sense is dynamic, coming as it does from a nondual spiritual concept of the cosmos as a unified movement. Thus, healing is not a battle between disease and health (evil versus good), but is a restoration of intrinsically harmonious perspective. Within this orientation, relationship encompasses rather than distances, and right relationship is participation in a cosmic integrity expressive of dynamic well-being. Well-being is not defined through alienating standards but by participation in Beauty. As awareness of wholeness grows, so does the experience of well-being.

Conventional discussion of herbs is akin to talking politics, a realm in which one can become endlessly involved with what each candidate's policies are and how government will be influenced by them. There are all kinds of issues and strategies to ponder and engage with, but to focus on the paradigm itself is another matter. Engaging at this core level encourages transformative change, not just surface rearrangements.

In shamanic herbalism, plants are living allies with which to address primary stratas of awareness and response. Suppose you inquire about a medicinal herb in the same way that you might inquire about a human practitioner. To know the practitioner's attributes as a healer, you could ascertain that persons' "properties," regarding them, for instance, as the facts of her being of Hispanic descent, left-handed, strong, sixty years old, related to a lineage of healers, and possessing keen eyesight. Further, you might discern through experience that the practitioner has a gentle touch and a particular knowledge of the nervous system. These properties suggest possibilities about what the practitioner might be good at as a healer. On one level there is great relevance to these specificities; they are a language easily understood at the surface level. Moving to a deeper knowing of the practitioner through a different kind of discernment may reveal capacities primary and fundamental, capacities such as the practitioner's ability to listen and intuit, to focus and act in alignment with well-being. The engagement of these capacities with another in a healing relationship is a more subtle language. At the core level of discernment is the knowing that is unified relationship, a language so intimate it is an illumined silence.

The shamanic knowing of herbs is concentric, an understanding and employment of all three languages. It is tremendously useful and respectful to learn names, individual natures, and appropriate applications of medicinal plants. But that is not where knowledge and practice ends, or is centered, in shamanic herbalism. Form is an octave of consciousness. In actuality, any condition can be addressed with any herb, or no herb, using that most primary of healing languages: resonance based on alignment with well-being.

This book is a sharing of both traditional knowledge and personal experience. Consensus about how to do things or how to interpret information is not what unifies shamanic practitioners; fierce debate (or good-natured acceptance of differences) characterizes most esoteric discussions, herbal and otherwise. What determines "correctness" in how plants are used is not subscription to a particular viewpoint; correctness is determined by the individual's depth of relationship with those plants, and the success of the application. The information in this book is derived from a time-honored approach to herbs—that of direct alliance within a continuity of ancestral wisdom. What emerges from that approach is, to a certain extent, idiosyncratic, but that uniqueness speaks to the truth of resonant relationship, and as such can be regarded as an encouragement, not a disclaimer. For however much is already known about herbs, there still awaits the uniqueness of your living truth of relationship. May your journey be one of great discovery and healing.

PART I

SHAMANIC HERBALISM

Wise folk say, every beginning
implies an ending.
Not quite so, say the trees
as leaves drop from visible splendor
to the hidden roots they nourish.
While snow-quilted branches dream,
all is renewed.

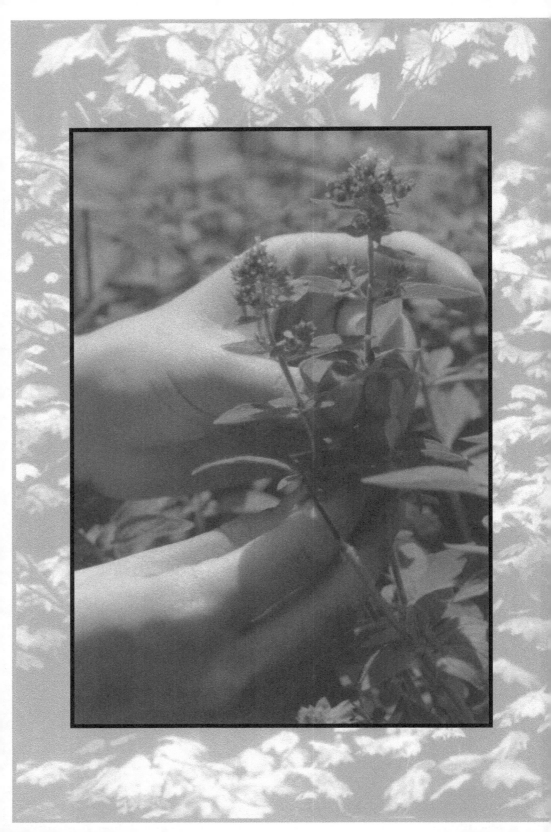

Chapter 1

Gathering and Growing Herbs

My canoe rounds a bend in the quick-flowing, slender river, and I see that the facing bank of the next curve is lined with a dense patch of blue vervain. I let the boat drift, the current carrying it to the vervain's embankment, nestling the boat into the shore's embrace.

Morning sun reclines on leaves and water. I bring out my tobacco pouch and make an offering to the river and the vervain, and to the beauty of the day. Then I harvest. The vervain is plentiful, but I don't need to take much. I lay the cut herbs in the bottom of the canoe and cover them with my jacket. A feeling of blessing flows from the river, the sun, and the fertile earth through the vervain, returned to the cosmos through my grateful awareness of its gifts. From the vervain's leaves will come teas and extracts that calm anxiety. The medicinals will carry the peaceful vitality of river, sun, earth, and morning breeze, and the joyful gratitude of the harvester—all entwined with the herb's physical virtues.

Another moment beckons. It is May. My son and I drive across the western states, on our way to Michigan. Each night we set up our tent in a different state park. On a country road in eastern Washington we spy wild roses blooming beside a field, and stop to gather some.

The air around the roses smells pink. We are entranced by the fragrant profusion of flowers. After making a prayer and offering we pick blossoms—never too many from each bush. They are fairy things. Our hands move tenderly; the petals feel like butterfly wings.

The next day, in the high plateaus of Wyoming, we stop for prairie sage. The air shimmers with heat, though it is early in the day. Sagelands stretch confidently beneath a cloudless sky. I feel the presence of rabbits, eagles, snakes, coyotes, hawks, and small lizards, their lives woven with the sage's. We harvest, then retreat to the car. Sage leaves join rose petals in the backseat, spread across paper to dry.

That night when I unzip the tent to go to bed I see my pillow covered with roses, and my son's pillow covered with sage. After gently scooping the herbs into bags, we find that the pillows are permeated with the scents of wild roses and prairie sage. We sink through the fragrant mist into beautiful dreams.

The attention you bring to the gathering of herbs can be a significant aspect of your relationship with plants, creating continuity and integration. Personal awareness of a plant's origin, the context of its organic life, and the circumstances of its harvest combines knowledge and participation in a way that powerfully informs your work with that plant.

When I see children (some of them adults now) whose births I attended as a midwife, I feel a unique knowing of them. I will look at Solomon, perhaps, and remember the summer heat of his natal day—the way he opened his eyes and gazed at me with his head in this world and his body in his mother's. Or I may see Sarah and recall the blizzard that gave way to a moon-washed midnight silence waiting for her emergence, which came with the rosy dawn.

It is likewise with gathering plants. There is something of the moment's circumstance that fixes itself within the harvester and harvested, influencing your perception of the plant and manifesting in your work with it. When you keep this in mind, it helps you remember to gather herbs in an attentive and joyful way. When you harvest you want to include, not sever, the larger context of energies that created and sustained the life of the plant. The gathered herbs are more potent when you have not separated them from their natural and spiritual connectedness to life's web. The more you do your harvesting in this way, the more wonderful you feel about the herbs you gather and the better they feel about your use of them. It is an intangible, though sensible, truth of relationship.

It is much easier to discern appropriate application for parts of a plant if you have seen the whole plant alive in its natural habitat; the recollection of seeing a delicate orchid or a robust burdock is more evocative than the sight of a jar of herbal capsules. It can be challenging to regard a powdered substance as a sacred being with unique, memorable attributes—imagine the difference in your response between seeing a magnificent redwood tree and seeing a pile of redwood sawdust. If you have never seen a redwood tree, you might have difficulty connecting the sawdust with a specific, embodied spirit. By developing familiarity with living plants and having meaningful occasions when harvesting them, you also develop understanding and appreciation. Abstractions become vital experiences.

It is late spring on the Washington coast. I carry baskets under my arm, scissors and tobacco pouch in hand. The woods are a tangle of salal and rhododendrons between madrone and fir trees. They open into a clearing—ground disturbed during logging. The nettles here, which I have come to harvest, have astonishing height and are intensely green. Encountering a force field of herbal energy, I abruptly stop and set down the baskets. I gaze at the grove of nettles, awed by their vigor. I sing to them—spontaneous admiration. I gather the leaves from the smaller plants cautiously but intimately, using scissors and bare fingers, occasionally reaping a sting along with a leaf. I don't mind the sting—during the following days it is a reminder of the nettle's medicine of guardianship over disturbed land: good medicine. I use the leaves in an iron tonic for pregnant women. As I harvest, I tell the nettles that their virtues will become part of new life in the endless cycle of birth and transformation.

The principles for gathering wild plants are commonsense tenets of right relationship. Take only what is needed, certainly no more than twenty-five percent of a grouping of plants, and never harvesting endangered species. When collecting bark, be sure not to girdle trees by stripping all the way around any portion of the trunk. Harvest in a way that enhances future plant growth by scattering seeds or spores, cleanly pruning leaves or branches, filling in holes you dig. Have care for the habitat.

Gather plants in places free of pollution, evolving a reverent manner of interaction in whatever way is natural and sincere for you. Remember that your state of mind influences what your hands touch. Gather in accordance with the season and time of day appropriate for harvesting various plants and plant parts: leaves are picked before or after the plant flowers, in morning or late afternoon; flowers are gathered early in their blooming, in the morning; seeds are harvested when fully ripe; roots and bark are collected in early spring or fall, at midday or evening.

Plants not used fresh should be spread or hung to dry in warm, airy places, out of direct sunlight. The drying plants should not be exposed to temperatures beyond 95 degrees (115 degrees for roots). Roots must be cleaned and cut for efficient drying. In whole or cut form, leaves retain potency for six months to one year; roots and bark for two to three years. In powdered form the potency of an herb is greatly reduced, giving a shelf life of about two to three months, though herbs like cayenne and goldenseal maintain efficacy longer. Most dried herbs are best stored in glass and kept away from light, moisture, and excessive heat.

Gathering wild herbs is one way to learn about and interact

with plants. Gardening is another. The tradition of gardening in accordance with moon cycles may appeal to you. During the waxing moons, plan and prepare your garden, and plant annuals or crops that bear their usable parts above ground. Prune at this time, if you hope to stimulate growth. Fertilizing, grafting, and making stem cuttings are also appropriate activities during waxing moon cycles. Harvesting, weeding, and pruning to discourage growth are done during waning moons. These are also advantageous times to plant root crops. When the moon is full, gather herbs or mushrooms that are to be used for esoteric or magical purposes.

Cultivate, weed, and gather plants during periods when the moon is passing through an Air sign. Moon in Aquarius is a good time for irrigation; moon in Libra is good for planting flowers, vines, and root crops. The ideal context for planting and fertilizing is when the moon is in a Water sign, particularly in Cancer or Scorpio. Pisces encourages root growth and propagation of aquatic plants. Plant herbs when the moon is in an Earth sign, especially ones whose medicines are concentrated in the roots. Cultivate or plow in Taurus; plant rhizomes or improve soil in Capricorn. During Virgo moons buy seeds, cultivate, make plans, tidy the garden, and give the plants attention. Fire signs favor clearing the garden sites and gathering; in Aries, harvest herbs and root crops. In Leo, weed and cultivate; and when the moon is in Sagittarius, plant onions, leeks, garlic, and chives.

Herbs can be interplanted with vegetables, shrubbery, and flowers, or grown in separate arrangements. You might choose to garden in a medicine-wheel configuration or a star-shaped pattern, a spiral design or a maze. The plants you invite into your garden will suffuse that space with their specific and collective energies in relation to the garden's design and the gardener's expressed intentions. The more focused and mindful you are in your gardening efforts, the more response you will notice from the plants. Direct communication and receptivity should not be overlooked.

It is early autumn and I am making tinctures for my son to take to college. I dig elecampane roots from my neighbor's garden. The plants are enormous. I love the fragrance of their roots. The elecampane will be combined with spring-tinctured mullein, the tops of which now reach the eves of my house, and with osha and licorice roots, for a respiratory tonic.

My son is a lanky young man, over six feet tall, and the height of the elecampane and mullein plants reminds me of him. The strength of the mountain that these plants grow on will be carried by the tincture, accompanying my son to college and helping him stay connected with the mountain. I harvest with love for the elecampane, for the mountain, for my neighbor, and for my son. My hands touch cool roots in the secret depths of the soil.

Communication begins with the making of sacred space: in preparation of the soil, in cooperation with the land, in alignment of intention with well-being's larger design. A garden should emerge from, not be imposed upon, the ground. Listen to the advice of the elder beings—the trees and stones. Spend time with the land; know what abides there. Observe the land through at least one cycle of seasons before you bring forth your garden. Ask the land to describe its dreams in the language of vegetation.

The herbs you invite into your garden may come from cuttings, transplants, or seeds. The garden's hospitality should be nurturant and comfortable so that plants feel at home and will prosper there. You may want to put special stones or statues amid your mandala, or make offerings, prayers, and invocations as you form and tend your garden. I sing to seeds and pat the soil over them with the same respectful affirmation I would give children, recognizing their miracle and trying to serve their emergence and fruition.

One spring I was planting seeds, the soil still cool from winter's rest. I poked a finger into the sandy loam and a puff of light sprang forth as if it had waited in the dark ground for months, eager to rejoin the rising day.

That herb garden, in Michigan, was the setting for many nonordinary events. I have never worked with a space quite like it. My only encounter with a completely substantial-looking representative of the Little People occurred there. He was perhaps a foot tall, dressed in brown—including hat—and had a curling beard. Near the garden was a grove of trees I had deemed off-limits to human presence (except during Celtic holy days when I ventured to its center to place offerings). It was set aside for the sacred beings of the land—a way of remembering, and reminding others, that wild places belong to themselves and humans should reconsider their imagined right to tread wherever they please.

Another memorable experience happened the day after summer solstice one year. I was weeding in the herb beds when a great lassitude came over me. It was so compelling that I lay down in the path between the beds and drifted into a half-sleep. In that state I dreamed that I was in a deep forest, under a tree. I heard strange piping music. As the sound grew louder I saw living forms taking shape, materializing and then changing to other shapes and colors, as if brought into manifestation and transformed by the music. I felt a presence beside me and it seemed that I opened my eyes into wakeful observation, seeing a face with wide-set green eyes bending over me. A wash of vertigo jolted me into actual awakening.

I sat up feeling very dizzy. The world pulsated. I went into the house, my head throbbing, and staggered to bed. During the night I dreamed a volcano erupted through the middle of the house. Morning brought reorientation, though a strangeness lingered. In later years I dreamed of Pan several times, receiving esoteric teachings from him. That alliance is one I approach with great care.

The design of an herb garden can influence experiences had within it. Creative patterns are one of the delights of gardening. A planned herb garden can be like a ceremony, formalizing your intentions and actions within a designated structure. My herb beds in Michigan were outlined with field stones in

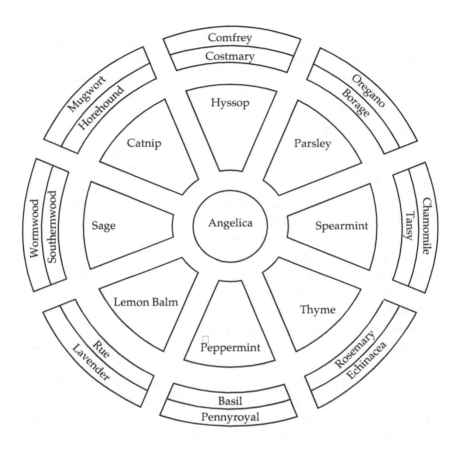

an octagonal design. This pattern was representative of the eight Directions—cardinal points and cross-quarters of the compass— forming a medicine wheel, with angelica in the center for spiritual grounding and guardianship. Working in this garden in awareness of the pattern's significance and the energies attracted and transmitted by the activated design and the herbs was movement in a sacred space. It was a reminder that simple daily tasks can be sacred and powerful, and can be accomplished in an atmosphere of respect, mindfulness, and joy. The work becomes a participation in healing—a world work—connected to the web of life on many levels, as my experience with Pan suggests.

Connection extends through the material planes as well. An organic garden has more than plants in it. It has bugs, worms, mammals, birds, reptiles, amphibians, and other creatures trafficking through, integrating with the larger ecosystem. One of my favorite garden denizens was a gigantic toad. A garter snake used to curl under a calendula bush to watch me water my garden, until I absentmindedly turned one day and blasted it with my hose. Despite my remorse, the snake did not come back. The life in your garden teaches you about interdependencies and relationships, and this becomes part of your knowledge of herbs and their medicines.

By kneeling in sunshine, planting, weeding, watering, mulching, harvesting, admiring, you learn the details of green life. Your hands smell of plant magic, your mind's eye holds images of stem, leaf, flower, and seed, unfolding in the light. The more you know a plant's textures, fragrance, color, flavors, and patterns of form and growth, the deeper your understanding of its gifts. The more you observe a plant's role in the health of its habitat, the clearer is your realization of its contribution to well-being. Your understandings and realizations in these realms are your guides in using herbs. The plants speak not only in the language of their individuality but in the vocabulary of larger context. Gathering and gardening are two ways to learn the healing language of plants.

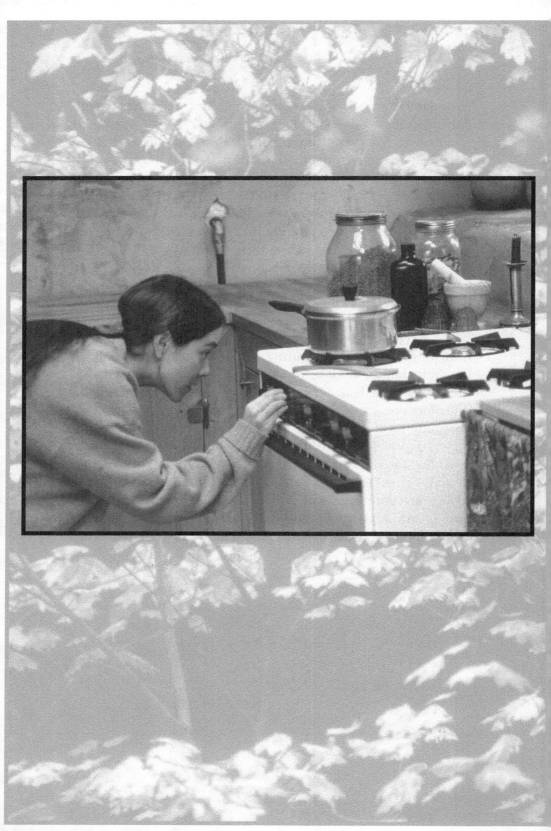

Chapter 2

Preparing
Medicinal Remedies

When applying herbs medicinally you choose from an array of preparational forms, each form having corresponding conditions for use. Your selection may be based on intuition, on conventional herbal protocols, or on what is at hand.

At the time of harvest you may have known the specific use you planned to make of a plant and, if so, communicated that plan to the herb. Whether or not you did that, the time of preparing a remedy is an opportunity for prayer and communication.

I am at a birth. The scene is peaceful—labor is going well—but I feel nauseous. I ask the laboring woman's husband if there are tea herbs in the house, and he names what they have. When he mentions comfrey something in me responds affirmatively, though comfrey is not specific for nausea. In the kitchen I pour a handful of the dried leaf into my hand as I wait for the water to boil.

"Sacred comfrey," I say to it, "I need your help. I ask you to influence my solar plexus, bringing calmness, clearing away illness, so I can fully attend to this birthing. Thank you."

I cover the herb with my other hand and attune my awareness to the comfrey. When I feel a clear sense of its spirit I align with that medicine—an inner prayer on an unspoken, energetic level of communication and partnership.

When boiling water is poured over the comfrey, its color and fragrance are released. I sit cradling the cup of steeping tea between my hands, closing my eyes and breathing the comfrey's signature aroma—an enveloping, stalwart presence. After drinking the tea my nausea disappears and does not return.

Selecting appropriate herbs and forms of application is only one aspect of medicinal preparation. Explicit, expressed intention and alignment with universal harmony are also important. This is part of the difference between the work of shamanic practitioners and other sorts of specialists. A shamanic healer is aware of and engages subtle forces. Prayer, ceremonial actions, and other spiritual procedures are ways the healer accesses the state of mind needed to perceive and interact with those forces.

Efficacy of approach depends on using procedures that work, not on adopting any particular set of ritual protocols. As I make a tincture, decoction, poultice, or whatever, I find it useful to name and visualize the person I am preparing the remedy for and to talk to the herbs about who the remedy is going to. As in the example about the comfrey tea, I also describe the condition or situation that has instigated the remedy's preparation. This gives clarity and focus to my actions and infuses the herbs with specific intentions. Further, it engenders an atmosphere of cooperative effort.

A pregnant woman comes to me wanting a home birth, but because she has genital herpes her doctor considers her a candidate for cesarean section. The herpes lesions have been active on and off during the pregnancy.

It is decided that if there comes a point close to term when the lesions retreat and blood titres are satisfactory, I will attempt to induce labor for a home birth. Such a point does come. We agree that if nonaggressive prompting of labor does not succeed, there will be no pushing into riskier, more invasive techniques.

Earlier in the pregnancy I made a tincture from blue and black cohosh roots and small amounts of spikenard, ginger, and licorice roots. When it comes time to try inducing labor, I hold the tincture bottle and make a prayer that the herbs bring on labor if it is a right and healthy thing to do. Several hours after the tincture is given the labor begins, and proceeds quickly and smoothly into birth. There is a feeling of harmonious consensus among all participants: herbs, mother, midwife, baby, and—from a distance—doctor.

I always carried herbs in my birth kit, mainly in extract or tincture form. Nestled against my fetoscope, cord clamps, bulb syringes, gauze pads, and other midwifery paraphernalia, they took on the aura of that world of sleepless nights, measured breathing, patient courage, womanly and womb-ly fluids, and transformative emergence. Where you keep your herbs influences their energies and is a facet of your relationship with plants. Respectful handling of ceremonial or healing herbs does not begin during ceremony. What happens in the daily affairs of your household, in the way you store and prepare herbs, and in the company they keep all affect the herbs' total beingness. The herbs in my midwifery kit or the sacred plants in my medicine bag partake of whatever energies share those containments, and in turn affect the bags and their contents.

Tools and vessels used to harvest, store, and prepare herbs should be mindfully chosen. In strengthening your connection to plants you may find it beneficial to use as much direct contact as possible, rather than employing intermediary implements. Handwork is often slower, more interactive, and more painstaking than machine or tool use, and for those reasons is more conducive to the cultivation of awareness, alliance, and power. If you use tools such as knives, scissors, shears, mortars and pestles, and so on, you may want to set aside consecrated or smudged (cleared) implements that are reserved for healing or ceremonial work with herbs. Those don't have to be fancy tools—their specialness comes in how you regard, maintain, and use them.

The process for making herbal remedies involves heating; cooling; adding or evaporating water; combining herbs with alcohol or oil; maceration; extraction; and other alterations, transformations, and blendings. All of these are elemental processes. In carrying them out you are inviting the herb on a journey that takes it far from its original life and form. You invoke the irrevocable forces of fire, water, earth, and air, to shape an opportunity for healing.

As you make your herbal remedies, think of your kitchen as a temple or medicine lodge. Attune to an herb's spirit, perhaps hovering beside you, as you take the herb's fresh vibrant leaves and pour fired water over them, releasing vapors that rise through your subconscious, whispering of light, mist, spring breeze, steady Earth, and the beauty of living beings. Heed that spirit at your side. Perhaps it will say, "You need more beeswax for that salve" or "Simmer that decoction a tad longer" or "Pay attention—that's my soul you are grinding so inattentively."

Your thoughts, intentions, emotions, degree of awareness, pace, and level of cleanliness all affect the remedy being prepared. Attuning to the herbs; expressing aloud your plans, desires, and gratitude; visualizing the well-being of the person the remedy is for; and moving with unhurried calm and present-mindedness are ways to keep yourself harmonious with the work of healing.

The use of fresh herbs is generally preferred, with some exceptions (goldenseal and yellow dock come to mind). If you are using dried herbs, store them in as whole a form as possible, waiting until you are preparing a remedy before crushing, grinding, or cutting the plant material. Potency is better retained in whole form.

If you obtain store-bought remedies or preparations made by other people, or buy the herbs you use for remedies, give these extra attention. The plants may have been harvested mechanically or unwisely, irradiated, sprayed, contaminated, mass-produced as a remedy, improperly stored, or otherwise maltreated. Wildcrafted and organically grown herbs are not immune to such misadventures. The following suggestions pertain to purchased herbs and packaged herbal remedies:

1. Use reliable, reputable sources. Know the origins of what you procure and the people involved. Know how to ascertain quality.
2. Check that what you receive is what you want. Plant identifications are not always accurately presented. For example, much of what commercially passes for skull-cap is actually germander. Learn Latin names in order to avoid confusion.
3. Dowse or hand-scan for vital energy. Attune to spiritual presence. Get an internal sense of yes or no about using a remedy.
4. Welcome the herbs that come into your home. Introduce yourself. Express gratitude for healing allies.
5. Smudge or otherwise clear purchased herbs or remedies. Repackage them if necessary, storing them in suitable containers and environments.
6. Consider potentizing the herbs or remedies with crystals or stones, or by placing them in proximity to altars or medicine objects.
7. Along with learning about their conventional attributes, explore what influences are carried by the herbs you are using before you actually ingest them.

 I make a tincture with a certain species of mushroom. For six weeks I watch the extraction process. The mushroom is one I have ingested but not one I have known to be tinctured. I strain the finished extract and hold the jar between my hands. An emphatic "NO!" reverberates through my mind. The tincture is immediately poured on the ground, with gratitude for the teaching.

Another time it is an invitation to knowing that I accept. I sit beside a garden nightshade, attending closely to its details of leaf, stem, flower, and fruit. I absorb all I can of what it expresses, and in turn offer respect and inquiry. It invites me to taste—not berry, but leaf—and I do, a cautious amount, chewed but not swallowed. It warms and slightly numbs my mouth. I thank the plant for this small knowing of it—the memory stays clearly: the white starlike flowers, the dark berries, the beckoning.

My husband and I are hiking in the woods behind our house. It is a forest I have lived in for eight years. We come upon a plant that has been dug up and gnawed on by an animal—from the signs, probably a raccoon. Neither of us recognizes the plant but decide that, if the animal found it edible, perhaps we will too.

We nibble a little of the exposed root, which is what the animal had been chewing, and resume our walk. After a few minutes I tell my husband that I feel funny. He replies, "I feel funny too." We walk some more. My mouth tingles, my nervous system tingles; I feel somewhat anesthetized. After a few more minutes I ask my husband if he knows where we are. The familiar forest does not look familiar any more.

My husband is an expert woodsman and has an uncanny sense of direction. He looks baffled. "I'm lost," he admits. I giggle. I can't help it—I feel funny. Neither of us is worried. After about twenty minutes the effects of the plant wear off, and it is obvious where we are and how to find home. Later, looking in texts, we tentatively identify the plant as May apple (also known as American mandrake).

While I am allergic to a plethora of drugs I have never been harmed by ingesting a plant, though certainly they are not substances about which to be cavalier. Very small amounts of certain plants can kill big, healthy people. Ancient herbal systems like that of the Chinese found ways of processing toxic herbs, such as aconite, so that they could be used medicinally. The art of preparing a remedy is one that understands the plant's attributes, and how to bring certain of those to the fore. What is drawn from an herb by a water base sometimes differs considerably from what is extracted by alcohol, for example. An inappropriate steeping time can empty an herb of its virtues, or fail to invoke them. Some herbs must be used fresh or in whole form in order to be efficacious or safe, and so on.

The shamanic herbalist learns those things from the plants and from other healers, past and present, gaining both knowledge and intuitive wisdom. Proper preparation of both practitioner and remedy opens the door for healing.

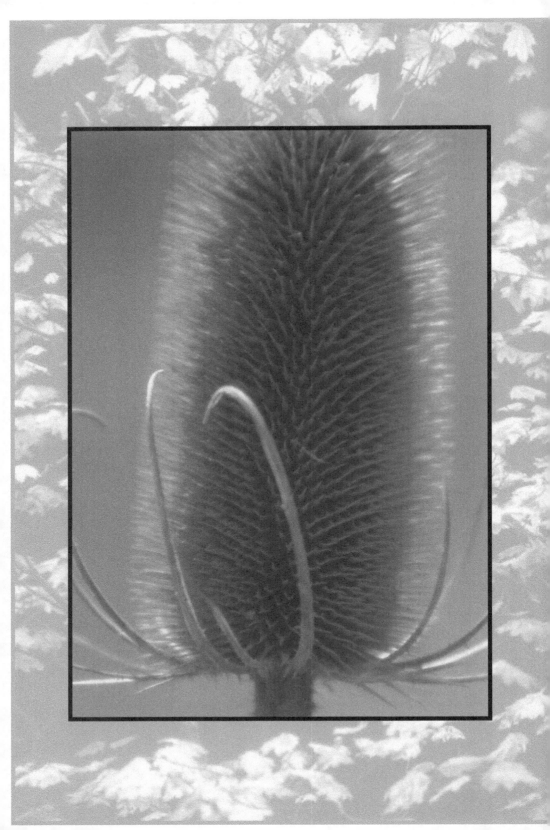

Chapter 3

Healing with Herbs

The first thing to consider when approaching herbs for healing is that plants were on the earth long before humans: they are not accessories to our tenure. This understanding is a reference point for respectful relationship with herbs.

To know a plant's healing attributes, a shaman does not analyze chemical constituents (though there is nothing wrong with doing this). Instead, the shaman sees the web in which the plant participates: the way the plant interacts with its habitat and all beings within that habitat, and the way the habitat interacts with the larger web of being.

That web's design is a complex, multilayered dynamic—a mandala of interdependent health. Each plant plays a role in the larger dynamic: perceiving the role gives insight into how health can be expressed in human interaction with the plant. That perspective is different from one that judges a plant's usefulness and application on the basis of human illness. Planetary health could be seen as a dance we do together, in mutual awareness and cooperation. This shifts the healer's point of view from user to partner and from illness to wellness.

Each plant has a unique vision of and contribution to wellness. The nettles' view of wellness, for example, is protective, strongblooded, empathetic, and rigorous yet nourishing. The lemon balm's, on the other hand, is calmly solicitous, cool, gentle, and assuring. When you perceive well-being through the perspective of a certain plant, you begin to know the plant's way of healing. Instead of looking for connections between disease symptoms and plant constituents, you attune to affinities between people's needs for perspective and plant's views of well-being. This is one way you can align with healing consciousness—it allows you to consider both plant and person in a wholeness of healthy, interdependent relationship.

Modern Western herbalism talks about a plant's properties. Chinese and Ayurvedic systems refer to a plant's energetic characteristics. Shamanism orients to a plant's medicine—its particular truth of being.

Truth of being, in plants, is explicit—there is no confusion of identity. Each plant is like an embodied idea: its medicine is a state of mind, a perspective of pervasive consciousness. When you partake of that medicine, you recall that perspective; you include, in yourself, that state of mind, which is then mirrored in your state of being.

A man comes to me who has smoked marijuana treated with a toxic chemical. He speaks of being ill for weeks, and of having trouble concentrating or maintaining a train of thought. His skin and eyes are jaundiced and he reports feeling depressed.

I give him an extract of milk thistle seeds. The seeds are very difficult to harvest; the work requires attention, patience, and perseverance—all the qualities this man is lacking. Seeds in general are regenerative and clearing. This man's imbalance, in which he has lost concentration and continuity, is directly addressed by the thistle's medicine.

The liver, organ of decision, expresses feedback to the man about his inattention to discernment. If the man listens closely to the thistle, he may hear its teachings of attentiveness, and in doing so, receive its healing gift of regeneration. He may align his self-perception with the thistle's outlook on well-being.

• • •

An herb will describe its truth on many levels accessible to human translation. It speaks to the eyes through its shape, color, growth configuration, and other details of appearance. It informs the subconscious through its odors. It offers the language of texture to the fingertips, membranes, and skin. It speaks evocatively through taste.

An herb expresses itself in subtle ways also, understood within psychic and spiritual receptivity. It offers the energies of its habitat, of its harvest and handling, and of the prayers and intentions with which it has been imbued. The plant releases its memories and the memories of its kind, and those also speak within the herb's medicine.

A woman who fractured her wrist is using comfrey to help its healing. Comfrey is a hardy plant: when you plow up a patch of comfrey it responds by increasing in numbers. Its perspective of wellness is proliferation of cells and knitting together that which is asunder. The fragrance of steeping comfrey is earthy, grounded. Its leaves are big; its aura is big; its pulp is fleshy, nutritive, and subject to quick decay. It speaks strongly to the human body: "Be here now. Be whole. Grow. Participate in life. Be part of things." The comfrey offers the partnership of its perspective to the woman who feels fractured, describing its vision of wellness in ways perceived through the senses, through the cells, through mind, emotions, and spirit. As the woman remembers her wholeness she manifests well-being—she heals.

Some schools of herbalism, notably that of Western naturopaths, see healing as a cleansing process. The focus is on ridding the body of toxins—purifying the blood, lymph, and colon by employing fasts, purges, enemas, and alterative herbs. Like allopathic medicine, it tends to create an adversarial relationship between body and mind. Shamanic herbalism centers on awareness and integration. It is a path of respectful mutuality, seeing all beings and all aspects of being as sacred and interconnected. Naturopathic approaches differ from shamanic perspectives in the same way religion differs from spirituality. The fixation on purifying, on exorcising the toxic sins harbored in the bowels, has a dogmatic and righteous quality to it. Shamanic herbalism, like spirituality, is less linear, less judgmental, more subtle and receptive, more encompassing. It sees healing as something that is realized within love.

Plants, for the most part being communal, often have natural affinities with other plants. Some herbs work especially well in tandem: echinacea and burdock, for instance, or comfrey and mint. You might think of them as dynamic duos—or sometimes trios or quartets and so on. They have complementary visions of wellness, each supporting, augmenting, harmonizing, or catalyzing the other's medicine. In order to heal with plants you must be sensitive to how and how not to combine herbs. The Chinese and Ayurvedic systems are especially expert in this. Many Western commercial formulations are not so soundly based. They combine herbs that are redundant or that distort or counteract each other's clarity of vision. Successful combining is a subtle art. Like a chorus of combined voices, the blended herbs should create moving, harmonious music that sings a clear, unified message to body and spirit.

In most combinations, as in most singing groups, there are one or two lead vocalists (primary herbs). Those are supported by the back-up singers (harmonizing, buffering, augmenting herbs) and carried by the bass rhythms of tonic herbs. The group is stimulated into really boogying by catalyzing herbs—the percussion section. A well-made combination will inspire the body to dance its way back into vitality and balance.

It must be remembered that shamanic herbalism is not a matter of prescribing a remedy for an ailment. It is a sensing of what human–herb partnerships will produce a complementary reality of well-being. Ten people with the same illness may need completely different remedies: the shamanic healer is not treating illness. A child's perspective or a pregnant woman's or a homeless person's all come from different contexts. What is needed for realization of health is referent to those individual contexts and outlooks, and to how those intersect with various plant outlooks.

I am at a spiritual gathering with thousands of other people. There is a communal food service, and something within it is malfunctioning—many people experience symptoms of food poisoning, myself included.

I go to the healer's station. It is a large canvas tent, dim and quiet inside. A woman sits on a stool and invites me to speak of what I'm experiencing. I say very little—there is a feeling of peace, centeredness, and direct understanding in the woman facing me, though she is obviously tired too.

We sit together for several minutes in attentive silence; she gazes at me, taking in what needs to be known. Then she nods and goes to her stores of remedies. She finds a small vial of homeopathic tablets and gives it to me. I know it is the right medicine. Our eyes meet as the vial passes from her hands to mine. She is a true healer. She listens to and "sees" each person coming to the tent—she does not mass prescribe a particular cure for food poisoning. After one dose of the tiny tablets, I am well.

Some people are more sensitive to plant medicines than others, attuning more easily to their messages. For example, I once opened a bag of lobelia, sniffed the herb's scent, and threw up. It was a response to its emetic medicine, not a reflex of sickness or distaste. On another occasion I took a sip of the tansy infusion a friend was drinking and started my menstrual cycle the next day, one week early. That kind of vibrational sensitivity means that some herbs should be used in very small quantities by such people, or in subtle forms. Instead of drinking an infusion, for instance, a footbath, sachet, or flower essence might be a more appropriate medium for alignment with a plant's medicine.

Other people are the opposite, requiring large quantities or frequent doses. A person might have a particular compatibility with water-based remedies, or with alcohol extracts, or with aromatherapy, and so on. The practitioner must discern not only the right plants to use, but the right form, amount, and rhythm for use. Some healers dowse with a pendulum or use kinesiology for this; some go by standardized protocols. Shamanic healers apply intuition, direct perception, spiritual guidance, and traditional knowledge.

How an herb is administered sometimes depends on less obvious underlying needs. Sometimes it is nurturance itself that is the healing vehicle. A person's core need may be to be touched, attended to, cared for. The plant's medicine, in that case, may best be received through massage oil, fomentations, warm teas, or other applications that emphasize comforting nurturance. Demonstrable love is the main ingredient in those remedies. Someone else may not need this, may not have caregivers to offer it, or may not allow time for doing it for themselves. Those people may be better served by an extract or homeopathic tablet, something easy and internally focused.

When people say, "I have trouble swallowing pills," it is often a signal that they are wanting some physical caregiving but have trouble asking for or receiving it. That tightness of inner conflict is as much in need of healing as the externalized imbalance presented as illness or injury.

It seems especially important that when children are feeling unwell they receive nurturant attention, not just curative substances. When that attention is given, children learn to nurture themselves, to choose healing allies that are nurturant, and to nurture others. This is one of the tremendous gifts offered by plant medicines, in contrast to allopathic treatments. Injections, harsh drugs, invasive and painful diagnostic procedures, and other modern medical processes strip away human dignity and reduce nurturance to a sympathetic smile from a nurse.

The ability to take care of oneself and others has become seriously impaired in modern life. The foods we eat, the fluids we drink, the ways our bodies are used or not used, the assaultive emotional and mental climate of the times, the substance abuse, and the dominant medical modes we turn to for "healing" reflect a profound loss of connection to nurturance and affirmative caregiving.

Renewing a respectful, engaged relationship with plants is a powerful aspect of planetary as well as personal healing. We trace the air we breathe, the food that nourishes us, the building and holding of soils, the cooling of ground and atmosphere, the source of shelter and medicine, the paper for this book, to plants. So many essential elements of survival and balance come from plants, yet those providers are taken for granted, demolished, abused, tampered with. Children (and adults) idly strip leaves, snap branches, and crush blooms underfoot in passing. Flowers are plucked for momentary pleasure or decoration. Lichens that spent years gaining fragile footholds on rocks are casually peeled off and destroyed by fidgeting fingers. Redwoods, fir, and cedars the vast, ancient likes of which we'll never see again are reduced to toilet paper and plywood pulp, and the natural communities they shelter are left in ruins.

So careless we have become with life, with what is sacred, with what is beautiful and irreplaceable, with our elders and healers, the rooted beings. The way we use herbs must embody reverence and awareness, otherwise it is merely another manifestation of a severed, consumptive perspective. It is our minds that need healing—our ways of living, seeing, and enjoining.

Each herb has a vision of life's goodness. Sit beside a plant. Make an offering and prayer; ask for understanding. Ask "What do you see, green being? What is the dream that rises through your roots from the wise, nurturant Earth; that sings through your stem, taking form in leaf, expressed in flower, tasted in fruit, preserved in seed; that reaches upward, trading secrets with the breeze; that whispers to birds and butterflies; that trusts its life to the process of each season? What do you know about well-being? What is your truth?"

Then listen—really listen—deep in the core of your resonance with well-being's truth. Each plant has a medicine song.

A friend comes to visit. She offers me a tincture of hawthorne berries, knowing my heart has been hurting. I take
it, though I usually make my own remedies. The tincture feels
right—I don't even read its label. I use it daily, and its effect is
immediately positive. Chest pain that stabbed for two years
becomes more intermittent, and after three months, disappears
almost entirely.

The tincture is labeled "Hawthorne Plus." The "plus" is
mostly *Cactus grandiflorus,* with small amounts of rosemary and
passion flower. The reading of those words gives me a surge of
joyful wonder. In my Florida childhood there was an occasion
when I was confined with illness—a dreary time, though it
probably did not last long in adult terms. One soft, tropical
night my mother took me for a drive along the Indian River.
The road was narrow and winding, edged by bending trees
bearded with Spanish moss. It was near midnight, much later
than I usually got to stay up, and it was just my mother and
me, another unusual event.

The rhythm of the winding drive was soothing. The river
breeze cooled and relieved the oppressive cling of illness. My
mother stopped the car and helped me out. The night was full
of insect songs and lapping river waves. The breeze hushed
through the old trees, stirring their mossy beards. My mother
led me to a tree—against it grew a cactus, and from the cactus
drifted a delicious fragrance, sweet and exotic. Turning on the
flashlight she'd brought, my mother directed its beam at the
single bloom on the cactus, the source of the wondrous emana-
tion. I was entranced.

The flower was brilliantly white—luminous, moon-white—
and huge, almost a foot across. My mother hoisted me to face it
at eye level, to breathe its vanilla-sweet exhalations. The flower
was, to me, a goddess. The magic of its perfume and glorious
yet secret blooming saturated my senses, suffusing my
imagination.

"Nightblooming cereus," my mother said, lowering me to earth again. "It fully opens at midnight—for one night only—then withers before dawn."

I never forgot. The magic of the flower stayed like a talisman from another realm, a touchstone throughout my life. When I learned herbalism I came across intriguing information about the medicinal uses of *Cactus grandiflorus*, a potent herb for heart ailments, but I did not know until reading the label on the tincture bottle that its common name is nightblooming cereus.

The rational, informational mind is a marvel of function, as useful to the shaman as to the scientist, but there are levels of activity that bypass the rational. They are like the dozens of jeweled spiderwebs that become visible in a field as the sun rises. The webs are there at other times, too, but are unseen. We walk obliviously past (and through) their lovely intricate embroideries. Shamans cultivate the seeing of such patterns—the perception of interconnected worlds threaded with life's shining strands. Through such mysteries healing moves, ruptures are mended, unions are reaffirmed.

Like plants we take root in purposefulness, and tend upward, seeking, growing. We express individuality, unfurl our leaves, flower in our efforts, bear the fruits of our actions, and encapsulate our hopes in the future's seeds. Like plants, each of us has a song to sing, a medicine, a dream of well-being that awakens in the light.

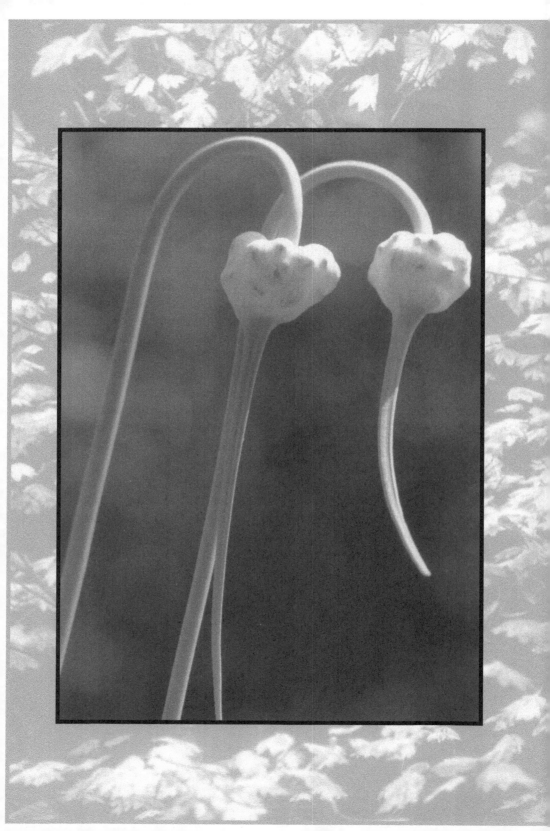

Chapter 4
Plant Allies

Traditional healers usually worked with a relatively small repertoire of herbs, using the herbs with which they felt aligned and which were available locally. Healers living in areas of profuse, diverse plant life, such as the curanderos in the jungle regions of Central and South America, had an especially large local inventory with which to engage. Regardless of how limited or extensive the resources are, there are always certain plants that call to a healer more than others.

Many modern herbalists, who now have global access to plants, unfortunately ignore common, local herbs in favor of whichever "celebrity" plants currently receive commercial acclaim. Even so, most herbalists are aware of their personal resonance with certain plants, and those herbs are especially relied on in times of doubt or crisis. They are the herbalist's solid, steady partners in healing, representing the essential connectedness a practitioner has with the green realm. It is possible that those plant allies are ones the practitioner has never seen in whole, living form, but more often they are ones the healer is familiar with through physical as well as abstract knowledge.

In addition to its physical appearance, the shamanic healer knows an ally's spirit form. Healers of that sort recognize when plant allies are present and are able to ask for an ally to be present when needed. A plant that serves as your ally or totem will make itself available in ways beyond the ordinary. At need, you may find it growing in unexpected places or during unseasonable times. It may offer extended or amplified potency, or make itself useful in ways not normally associated with its attributes. A little may go a long way.

When I gather plants considered special allies, I often choose times such as summer solstice, Lughnasad, or autumn equinox for harvesting. In doing this I honor both the occasion and the alliance, and feel a particular potency in the medicines made from those plants.

During herbal healings I often ask people if there are plants with which they have a special affinity and, if so, try to include those plants in what I am doing. I also find it useful to discern the possible herbal alliances of authors when I read botanical texts. Unless they are simply repeating knowledge gained from other texts, most authors of botanical texts reveal partialities to certain plants. When this is evident, I am able to get a better idea of the author's particular orientation. A "goldenseal" author is a different sort of person (and herbalist) than an "alfalfa" author, for instance. As well, listening to a person name and talk about plants he or she feels drawn to as we do healing work together gives unique information about the person's nature and his or her needs within healing.

Pondering your own plant affinities can render useful insights. During this process I ask questions both of myself and of the plant. The inquiry may go something like this:

> Where on the medicine wheel do I perceive this plant?
> What need is being addressed through my relationship
>   with this plant?
> What was my first encounter with this plant? What
>   drew me to it? What do I like about this plant?
> What are its predominant physical characteristics, and
>   with what do I associate them? What about myself is
>   like and unlike this plant, and how do I feel about
>   those parallels?

What has been my engagement with the plant? What
part has it played in my life? How have I used this
plant, and in what forms?

What is my sense of this plant's medicine? Where has
my information about it come from?

What is my relationship with this plant's habitat? What
does its habitat teach me about living and growing?

Some questions I lay before the plant may include:

What name do you prefer to go by? How shall I address you?

What is your work on Earth? What is your dream?
Your truth?

What teaching is offered through our alliance? What
medicine? What work can we do together?

What is your mirroring of me? What is the energy of
our resonance?

Are you an ally (short-term partnership) or a totem
(long-term partnership)?

What can I give you? What are the needs of your kind?

What am I not seeing?

Those sorts of questions deepen your perception of the plant
and expand your understanding of partnership. They create
a more participatory and purposeful relationship with the
plant, which manifests in positive ways through your healing practice.

If you have a number of herbal allies, you may want to consider the patterns revealed by those affinities, for instance, to
note whether the plants cluster in one Direction on the medicine wheel, all have the same color flowers, are used for similar
medicinal purposes, or have other repetitive characteristics.
Perhaps what will be notable will be a pattern of differences,
not similarities.

I am in a large midwestern city conducting a workshop about totems. One participant is a woman who calls herself by a tree name and claims the tree as her totem. It is a species of tree common to the midwest, and I ask her what has drawn her to adopting this tree's name. After several false starts, the woman admits she doesn't really know much about the tree. An admirable honesty compels her to add that she doesn't actually know what the tree looks like—she is simply attracted to the name.

While totem alliances require more than superficial connections, names are certainly part of a relationship. Conventional plant names run the gamut from romantic to ridiculous, but tracing the roots of those names can unearth worthwhile, interesting information. For example, mugwort was used as a beer additive (*wort*, from Old English, means "herb"); many other plant names imaginatively refer to characteristics of the plant's appearance, such as Dutchman's breeches or shepherd's purse. Such information furthers your understanding of herbs, and of human experience with them.

You may at times refer to a plant ally by a name that has personal meaning to you, or that has been provided by the ally. The herb may give you a song to use when invoking the ally during healing work, or when harvesting or planting.

Some herbs have traditionally been associated with certain animals. Sometimes the herb's association is incorporated into its common name, sometimes in folklore. Ground ivy is commonly known as cat's foot, for instance, because of the leaf's resemblance to feline paw prints. Devil's club, in northwest native lore, is an herb governed by the powerful spider spirit. Appendix 3 gives examples of herb–animal pairings, some more whimsical or obscure than others, and also lists herbs in relationship to their directional orientation on the medicine wheel. You may find this information useful for such things as assembling totem bundles or exploring alliance.

A one-winged crow living with my family is carried off in the middle of the night by a raccoon who tunnels into the crow's enclosure. The crow makes no sound, but I wake in the night, dragging myself out of a nightmare to find my husband also waking from a horrific dream. There is a sense of intrusion in the house, but my husband finds nothing amiss when he goes downstairs to investigate. In the morning we find two crow feathers, and the raccoon's tunnel.

I call a medicine man and ask him to look into the energies around our house: I don't tell him about the crow's abduction. The medicine man tells me a man opposed to the work I do is using a raccoon form to invade my space and cause harm.

I make a medicine pouch, filling it with herbs I associate with dogs; I add a tiny Rin Tin Tin figurine and the dog tag my last canine companion wore on his collar. I invoke dog energies into the pouch and hang it over our front door. There are no more intrusions.

A friend asks for a medicine bag imbued with the attributes of the East. I fill a small gold pouch with herbs correlating to the East and to Eagle medicine. As I put the herbs into the pouch a pinch at a time, I make prayers, asking for specific qualities of the East to be active in the presence of the herbs. The prayers clarify intention and focus its expression through a particular path of manifestation. I hold the filled pouch up to the morning sunlight, earnestly calling upon Eagle's medicine to empower the intentions now present in the herbs. As I do this, a bald eagle comes circling over the house, an affirmation of Spirit's continuity through all levels of experience.

Some affinities are not as pleasurable as others. At last count, my son has come into contact with poison ivy nineteen times. Though I traffic the same terrain he does, I have never shown signs of encounter with this warrior plant. My son even managed to acquire a poison ivy rash in the deep February snows of interior British Columbia one winter, while sledding alongside a warm-spring creek. His poison ivy tales convince even skeptics that supernatural relationships with plants are possible.

Having given some thought to this dance, my son feels that, despite its discomforts, his relationship with poison ivy is not an adversarial or negative one. What seems most amazing to me is that though he is observant, has lived in the woods all his life, and is quite intelligent, my son never knows when he's in the ivy.

Plant allies are teachers who do not always behave with the passivity expected of rooted, vegetative beings. Attitudes that emerge from the resource management perspective, the agricultural orientation, or the conquer-and-pillage mode all consider plants as things to be controlled or sacrificed in service to human desire and greed. Plants are generally regarded as having no sentient intentions of their own or no right to fulfill them. Those attitudes are both dangerous and sad. We can do much better in discerning a basis for relationship, and more truly benefit in the process as well.

When you respond to a plant as a kindred spirit, sacred alliance takes on the same reality as other sorts of partnerships. Feelings of real connectedness are what make the web of life come alive for you and be more than words and wishes. But plants—like people, animals, and mountains—do not always do what you want them to. They do not necessarily subscribe to your picture-book fantasy, or even to your pragmatic, sensible plan. Part of good relationship is acceptance of an ally's autonomous freedom of expression.

This is an important teaching for human beings, who are conditioned to see themselves as in charge and first in line. The teachings plants offer often times have to do with pride and presumption. Those are not the easiest messages to gracefully receive.

Certain plants and trees may play special roles in childhood or have particular and lasting significance to a group of people. Places you have lived or traveled are sometimes best remembered by what grew around them. Relationship with habitat is often defined through vegetation.

The community I stayed in for nine years in northern Michigan developed a tradition of plant kinship. My mother, a botanical enthusiast like her mother, began pairing people and plants. She had a knack for this and people trusted her views of them. At community meetings she read her lists of people–plant pairings; people laughed or blushed or nodded, sometimes requesting explanation but most often not. When babies were born, my mother observed them for some months or years, then announced their plant companions at a potluck supper or community gathering.

When I recall those people I still think of their companion plants, and vice versa. It made the community bigger, having the plants included, and it gave people a realm to consider if they chose to—a garden of discovery in themselves that was contiguous with a larger vision of community life.

There are many doors into plant alliance. One may open during a wander in the woods, or while perusing an herbal text, or in the midst of a vision quest, or out of a dream, or when sipping a cup of tea. Those doors may lead into expanded experiences of healing and realization.

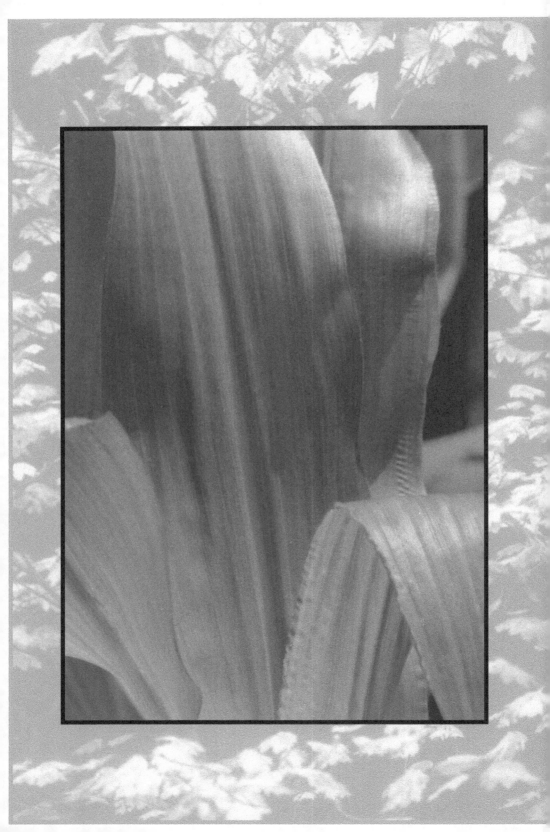

Chapter 5
Offering Herbs

One of the first things conscientious parents try to teach children is to say thank you for what is given. As children grow, they may also learn the second level of gratitude's teachings, which is to give in return. Without gratitude and reciprocity, our balances are lost on all levels of experience.

Life on Earth naturally moves in the round: seasons turn; what was sown is reaped. The web of life functions through a continuous, complex flow of give and receive. When too much is taken or when something is taken wrongly, without respect or wisdom, the entire web suffers. Witness what the destruction of the buffalo did to the life of the prairies. The newspapers today predict the same fate for the salmon within five years. Those are losses that are forever, losses that break the round of give and give back and rupture the web of life.

The use of offerings can be a way of remembering that we are part of a vast and sacred dance. Offerings enjoin us to look into the eyes of our partners and ask for a turn around the circle together. Making offerings is one way to clearly and humbly express intention.

When offerings are used in a focused, heartfelt manner, they are more than symbolic gestures. They actualize continuity, perpetuating and nourishing the integrity of life's wholeness. Offerings do not pay for something—nothing can buy life, and anyway there is nothing we own that is not a gift, bestowed upon us by that which creates being. Offerings honor the recognition of the transfer and remind us to participate in movement that is vital to life's balances, the rhythm of the round.

Offerings that are rote or self-conscious performances lack power, and yet, like recalcitrant children, we should still go through the motions of "please" and "thank you" because they are basic practices of community. At some point, lessons may come to life in a beauty of connectedness, in a reality of interdependency.

I am in England, at an ancient sacred site called Glastonbury Tor. It is a rounded, high, treeless hill standing amid a flat plain. Few people are here on the early morning of my visit. I climb the long, contemplative flight of stairs to the top and find a private place to pray and meditate.

Afterward, preparing to descend, I take a plum from my pocket, eating it as I begin the long walk down. I scan the ground for a small stone to take home to a friend, and when I see the right one, the reflexive gesture of offering is to lift the pebble and replace it with the clean-sucked plum pit and a murmured thank you.

I examine the pebble as I descend the stairs, then pocket it. A few visitors greet and pass me, going up. At the base of the tor I suddenly realize that my hat is missing from its securely clipped position at my belt. Immediately I know the reason, and I know where it is—unless the newcomers have already picked it up. The tor has given much to me that morning. During my prayers I am attentive and genuine in my offerings, but in taking the stone I am not, and I know better. The plum pit is convenient, though my gratitude is real.

I sigh, eyeing the steep, hot climb, feeling my hungry stomach, and wondering if the merry folk I've passed on the stairs are already exiting down the far side of the tor with my hat. Up I go again, and am given the grace of finding the hat where it dropped, beside the plum pit.

• • •

There are two plants frequently used as offerings in North America. The first is corn. Corn speaks to us of an ancient way of life. Its roots go deeply into native history in the Americas. In using corn as an offering and sacred plant, you link yourself to, and honor, that ancient relationship with corn or maize.

Corn is an androgynous plant, though it is often referred to as Mother or Grandmother Corn. It has male, pollen-producing flowers that grow on the tassel and female flowers, lower on the plant, that receive the pollen. Kernels then grow from the female part of the plant, becoming the corn's milky ears.

Through partnership with Native people corn went through profound changes, from a wild grass that self-seeded to a cultivated grain whose seeds are now encased in husks, dependent on human help to find their necessary placement in soil. The first offering of corn was to nourish, but for people to reap the nourishment they had to learn right relationship—how to properly care for the corn. In its altered form it was not possible to simply take the grain and wait for plants to produce more. Principles of respectful reciprocity, then, were the second offering of corn.

Through time, ceremonial traditions evolved that kept corn in the central position still seen in the regard shown this plant by the Hopi, Navajo, Pueblo, Cherokee, Iroquois, and other tribes. The sacred gifts of corn are still alive and being shared.

Ceremonially and as an offering, corn is used in all its forms: whole ears, seeds, pollen, meal, and cooked breads. The silk, husks, cobs, and other parts are used in many ways also, similar to the relationship the Plains tribes had with buffalo, the Northwest coastal people with salmon, and the Subarctic people with caribou and reindeer. In all those relationships the teachings of reciprocity are embodied. Prosperity and abundance depend on mutuality, the law of the round.

The corn's golden pollen, from the male flowers, carries life in a subtle yet potent form. It is a rarefied energy, used as food for spirits and totems—an offering that crosses between the worlds, almost etheric in its fineness. It enables nourishment's substance to manifest. The pollen is an initiator sparking a cycle that brings life's intention into form's expression. It is the inspiration catalyzing creative action. And the corn, in pollinating itself, reveals wholeness—it is complete, yet interdependent.

The corn's kernels can be any of the medicine wheel's directional colors: blue-black, red, yellow, or white. Sometimes a mix of colors is present on one ear, an example of harmonious diversity. Cornmeal, usually blue or various shades of yellow, is a familiar sight in many ceremonies. It is used for prayer, invocation, delineating sacred spaces, or gift offerings.

The meal is the corn's preserved nourishment. It sustains the people's bodies relative to the Earth's body. Its sweet substance nurtures life's form. In Cherokee stories, Corn Mother feeds the people from her own body—she *is* corn, and it is from the female part of the plant that kernels grow.

Corn as an offering is a recognition of principles of respect and reciprocity fundamental to sustainable well-being. Corn carries firm truths of good relationship: integrity, generosity, and mutuality.

The second plant frequently used as an offering is tobacco. Though there are indigenous tobacco plants in the Americas, the tobacco usually cultivated for smoking was originally an import. Tobacco is a beautiful, impressive plant. In considering its sacred use, it is inevitable that consideration must also be given to its abuse. Many people avoid tobacco in their spiritual practices because of negative or ambiguous feelings about the plant or the influences surrounding it.

It is predictable that anything of power will be prone to misuse. Tobacco, like corn, is a teacher of right relationship, though a teacher of a different kind. If you abuse your relationship with corn, it withdraws. If you abuse your relationship with tobacco, it overwhelms. There is no evil in the plant; tobacco is a mirror. It points out our own self-delusions and confusions. It reveals our self-doubts and vulnerabilities. Advertisements for tobacco emphasize sexiness, confidence, independence—all elusive qualities attractive to people beset by anxiety and feelings of inadequacy. The teenager population is a prime market.

I was a heavy smoker for nine years, quitting in my early twenties when I began practicing meditation. At the time I quit I was smoking three packs a day, much of it a custom blend of tobacco and hashish. I quit in the middle of a pack, in an unpremeditated moment of decision. Years later, through working with a Native American medicine man, I discovered a more positive relationship with tobacco.

In bedrock truth, I have never seen anyone who uses tobacco both habitually and ceremonially maintain a healthy dual relationship with tobacco. I say this without judgment, simply as observation. This subject will be touched on again in chapter 9.

Using tobacco as an offering herb is a form of use that, while not necessarily linked to smoking, is still inseparable from the corporate world of tobacco production. Unless you grow your own tobacco, or receive tobacco from someone growing it in a sacred manner, you are supporting a corrupt industry.

Some companies, make an effort to supply tobacco that is unchemicalized, and market their product in a straightforward way. (American Spirit is one such company.) As a practitioner, I frequently receive tobacco from people requesting ceremonies or medicine work. The tobacco is usually one commercial brand or another; when accepting it, I try to focus on the intentions of the giver and on the spirit of the herb.

If I am the one offering tobacco, I try to use homegrown plants, or brands such as American Spirit or Drum. Regardless of where the tobacco comes from, I clear it and pray with it before using the herb as an offering. There is no simple path to follow in reaffirming the sacredness of this plant in the midst of modern drug-consumer / drug-merchandiser consciousness.

Tobacco's medicine as an offering is resonant and full. It carries prayer and intention and thus is a teacher about truth and clarity of expression. Some stories say tobacco was the plant who volunteered to replace blood sacrifices, and in this we again hear principles of right relationship.

Tobacco is put into prayer ties for sweat lodges, vision quests, and other ceremonies. It is part of what is given to medicine people when asking them to do healing work, share their songs, answer questions, and so on. It is often the central herb in pipe ceremonies and is used, like cornmeal, as a prayer offering or embodiment of gratitude.

Other herbs can be called upon for those things, in accordance with what feels appropriate within your own understanding. I sometimes work with a variety of herbs for offerings and medicine bundles: sage, pine, sweetgrass, roses, lavender, and cedar. I carry herbs almost every time I go out of the house, keeping small packets of tobacco and sage in my coat pockets, purse, medicine bag, and truck's glove box. There are many spontaneous occasions for their use: special encounters, moments of prayer, opportunities for insight. The more you work with offerings, the more you realize how meaningful is that dimension of interaction. It takes things beyond a fleetingness of thought or emotion and suggests how Spirit can move on many levels, including the physical. Offerings indicate a path of integration. They invite direct connection with pervasive consciousness. Giving and receiving offerings unfolds spiritual participation.

 A Native medicine man agrees to be my spiritual mentor. He asks that I bring kinnikinnick when I next visit. There is a trading post fifty miles from where I live, but they are out of kinnikinnick for several weeks. Finally able to buy some, I again visit my mentor. I explain that I waited for the herbs to be in stock and that's why so much time has passed since my initial visit. The medicine man laughs and shakes his head. "You should've come over anyway," he says.

I am struggling with illness and feel drawn to asking help from a famous Native healer who lives a thousand miles away. I prayerfully assemble a blend of traditional smoking herbs, put them into a beautifully crafted deerskin pouch, write a brief but heartfelt letter requesting the healer's help, and send them off. I get no reply.

These two accounts of making offerings illustrate a range of responses found even within similar traditions. From the first medicine man I learned that giving is important, but form is sometimes secondary to other priorities. From the other medicine man I learned to pay more attention to what others truly need or find appropriate as offerings, and to not suppose my priorities to be theirs.

After six years of association, my spiritual mentor, who has diabetes, comes to my cabin with a pouch of tobacco mixed with bearberry. He offers it and asks if I will conduct a healing sweat for him. I accept the pouch, startled at this shift in our relationship. I feel unready, but not unable, and prepare diligently for the ceremony. Sometime during that process, tentativeness and self-doubt pass, leaving a clarity of practice. The herbs are used, and the gift of recognition remains to guide me.

A woman comes to one of our open sweats She is the wife of a Native ceremonial leader. The tobacco offering she hands me is tightly sewn into a small leather turtle; the turtle is painted with intricate symbols. Sometime after the sweat, I decide to put the turtle into an empty bird's nest perched about seven feet off the ground. Weeks later, when I check the nest, the turtle is gone.

These two stories of receiving offerings also show a range of experience. The offering from my mentor brought movement from egoic concerns to a larger spiritual identity. The turtle offering demonstrated movement wherein I understood how to be a bridge, not a destination, for offerings.

The ways of giving and receiving offerings are individual

matters, though if you participate in Native ceremonies you will find protocols to inform you. My friend Lawrence told me of a Native doctoring ceremony he attended. The people to be doctored, including Lawrence, made and brought tobacco ties to be used by the medicine man during the ceremony. The offerings were tiny, as is often the case for ceremonies using lots of ties. Lawrence thought his were small, but when placed next to the others his appeared conspicuously large.

As the ties were arranged together, Lawrence overheard the medicine man's helper inquire as to whether the medicine man thought the big ties were going to be workable. The healer, patiently arranging them with the others, replied with gentle confidence, "Well, we'll just give them a try."

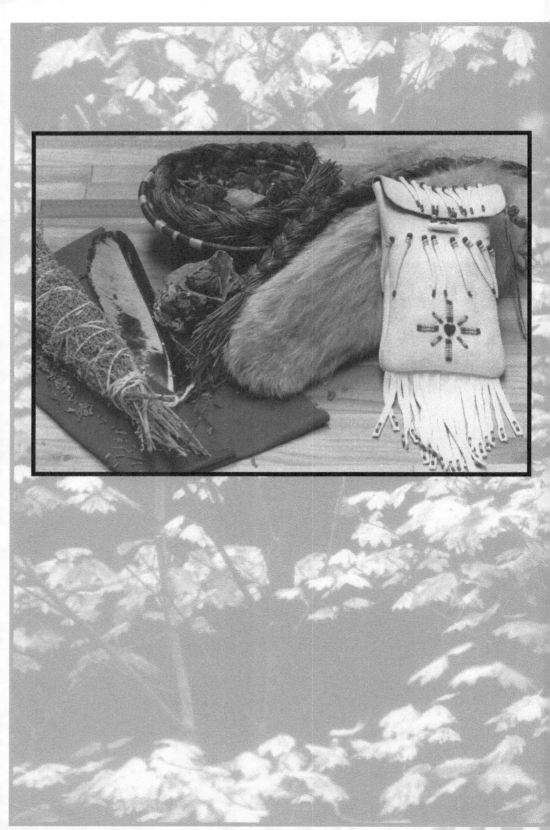

Chapter 6
Smudge Herbs

Smudging or censing is the practice of using smoke from smoldering plants to rid a person, place, or object of undesirable influences, or to attract beneficial presence. Many spiritual and religious traditions use some form of smudging. In North America there are six indigenous plants most known for this purpose.

The first herb I usually turn to as a smudge is prairie sage (*Artemisia tridentata, A. californica, A. ludoviciana,* and other sagebrushes). It is my first choice, partly because I live in the West, where sage is easily found and where, in working with it, I become more closely linked to my habitat, and partly because I feel an affinity with it. Sage's fragrance immediately calms and brings focus.

Prairie sage thrives in dry climates and poor soils. It is a hardy plant, withstanding bitter winters, scorching summers, and tearing winds. Its leaves are small and gray-green, and are either wrapped with string and dried while still on their twigs to create smudge wands, or stripped from their stems when dried and used loose. Sage wands are helpful for smudging large areas, when you want a lot of smoke for an extended duration. The dried, loose leaves are appropriate for most other circumstances. Air is a pervasive element—a little smoke goes a long way.

Sage is best gathered in spring, before it flowers. Properly dried and stored, its pungent, pleasing aroma stays strong for at least a year, then gradually fades. I find sage to be an ally who disperses negativity, guards sacred space, and allows spirit presences to be more readily discerned. Its fragrance is sharp, yet reassuring, centering, and welcoming. On occasions where it cannot be burned, you can crush sage leaves and rub the herb's essence over yourself or over an object needing clearing.

Another kind of sage, *Salvia apiana* (white sage), is also used as a smudge. It is related to garden sage *(S. officinalis)*, which is a transplant to this continent. The leaves of white sage are similar in texture and shape to those of garden sage. *Salvia apiana* grows in hot, dry climates; I have found it in southern California and Baja, though I have heard it also grows on the Minnesota shore of Lake Superior.

White sage has an acrid, pungent scent when burned. It is used to drive away intrusive influences or to purify ceremonial objects. Like prairie sage, it is sometimes bound into wands, or dried pieces of its pale gray, brittle leaves are burned loose. Though both plants are called *sage* and are used for similar purposes, the two herbs are different in character.

In areas where cedar grows, cedar foliage is burned as a smudge. Because of crossovers in common names, cedar is sometimes confused with juniper, which is also used ceremonially. The true cedars considered smudge herbs are mainly *Calocedrus descurrens* (California incense cedar), *Thuja occidentalis* (Northern white cedar), and *T. plicata* (Western red cedar).

Cedar trees are much revered by traditional Native people. The trees, when left to their natural cycle, grow very slowly and live a long, long time. I saw cedar stumps on Washington's Olympic Peninsula with six hundred to one thousand rings on them, each stump twelve to sixteen feet across. Few of those elders remain unlogged, though once there were many.

Cedar groves are quiet, beautiful sanctuaries. I once lived in one, an experience of introspective expansion. Those trees like to be near water—cedar's presence is cool, relieving, sympathetic. In winter, deer and bear often take shelter in cedar swamps.

Cedar's foliage is burned to clear away negativity and call in spiritual benevolence. Its scent is sweetly pervasive. Cedar smoke carries the prayers that are spoken in its presence. The smoke is traditionally used as a visionary medium during vision fasts by the native peoples of the Northwest, and green cedar foliage is sometimes laid on the heated stones inside sweat lodges. Cedar smoke, cedar foliage, cedar oil, and cedar sawdust all produce extreme allergic reactions in some people; thus, cedar should be interacted with carefully.

Cedar is mainly used as a smudge in the Northwest and Midwest, however the Native American Church's peyote ceremonies use cedar as their smudge, regardless of whether or not cedar is local to the ceremony's venue.

Pine is another tree whose foliage and resin is burned for smudging, though it is not as frequently used in that role as cedar. Pine is in the East on the medicine wheel. Its character is direct, vigorous, clear minded, and quick yet calm. Pine's medicine renews. Burned as a smudge, it is cleansing and carries intention.

Because pine is an evergreen, it is continuous in its availability and watchfulness, though like all plants it has cycles of growth, reproduction, and rest. Pine is the Celtic tree sacred to Cernunnos. It is a straight, strong tree, its needles sharp, but it embodies softness as well, a sense of kindness and peace.

The fifth plant encountered widely as a smudge is copal (*Bursera odorata*). Its resin is burned on coals to produce a heavy, sweet smoke familiar to Catholic churchgoers, since it is also used, combined with frankincense, as a religious incense. Many Native people of the southwest United States and Central and South America use copal as a clearing smudge. Its smoke is intolerant of negativity—it invokes order and spiritual priority. During winter I often set small chunks of copal resin on top of the woodstove in my house to begin my mornings. Being a resin, copal smudge resonates differently than leaf smudges; it has more of a dense, warming energy.

Last, but never least, is sweetgrass (*Hierochloe odorata*),

commonly called vanilla grass or Seneca grass. It prefers stream-
sides and marshes, appearing in the northern Great Lakes states
and some parts of Montana, Wyoming, South Dakota, Alberta,
and British Columbia. It is native to both Europe and North
America.

Sweetgrass is in the North of the medicine wheel: it is traditionally considered Grandmother Earth's hair and is braided
for ceremonial use. Dried, the plant has a lovely, graceful fragrance that remains almost indefinitely if the braids are properly stored.

Sweetgrass is an herb of blessing. Its smoke brings a sense
of well-being and ease. Smudging with sage is often followed
by burning sweetgrass. Shaved bits of the grass are ignited or,
more usually, the end of a braid is lit and the smoke gently
waved around people, objects, or spaces. Sweetgrass is sometimes burned during prayer to carry messages into the upper
realms.

Increased attention to the commercial value of sweetgrass
and its destruction due to habitat loss have endangered this
plant's survival in the wild. I recommend obtaining sweetgrass
from cultivated sources, conscientious wildcrafters, or your own
garden.

Athough smudging is a ceremonial act, it does not have to
be limited to formal occasions. Smudging is a good way to start
and end the day, and to care for yourself, your family, the spaces
you occupy, and the things with which you interact. It encourages prayer, healing, nurturance, attentiveness, and integration.
In a simple way, it expresses spiritual truth and power.

A letter arrives, loaded with hostility. Its recipient
smudges it with sage before opening it, and continues to
burn sage as she reads the letter.

Before leaving on a cross-country trip, I smudge the truck,
inside and out, speaking to the truck, the sage, and the
spirits as I work. As smoke curls around the tires, I pray for

guidance and surefootedness on the roads; as the engine is smudged, I ask for intelligent function and harmonious operation; reaching the bumpers, I pray for safe movement—no harm, no ill encounter. Inside the truck I give special attention to the driver's controls, the windshield and mirrors, and the space around the driver's seat.

A child has a nightmare and wakes crying. His mother comes in to soothe him. Before returning to bed, she smudges the child's room with sweetgrass. Its peaceful fragrance lingers through the night as the child sleeps.

A meeting takes place and those attending have diverse ideas. Before beginning discussion, everyone smudges with cedar, encouraging a feeling of receptivity and centeredness. Whenever conflict arises, the cedar is again turned to, restoring priority of purpose.

My son comes in the house, going directly to his room without speaking. The smell of sage drifts out his door. When he emerges, he is sad but calm. He has just come from discovering and burying a rabbit and goat who died from a neighbor's neglect and abuse. The scene he describes is ugly, grievous. After hearing his account, I smudge also, and make a prayer for the animals.

Dozens of examples come to mind: smudging can be an integral part of a practical, spiritual way of life. The herbs you are drawn to using and your sense of their medicines are aspects of ongoing relationship with plant allies.

Sometimes a feather or wing is used to direct smoke from smudge herbs; sometimes smoke is gathered and moved by the hands. Clay or stone bowls are traditional holders for smudge herbs. It is popular to use abalone shells to cup smoldering herbs, but some people, including many northwest Natives, consider it disrespectful to place fire within shells.

It is important to consider the implications of your chosen way of smudging. When you enact something calling on elemental forces and spiritual power you want to be clear about your core purposes and procedures. This begins with the formulation of intention, which arises from desire, understanding, and intuition. It is carried through in the herbs you choose, the surface you use for burning, and the way you ignite the herb and move the smoke. I was taught not to blow on smudge herbs. This is a teaching my own experience and feelings confirm. When smudging, I use the breath for prayer and let the herbs burn or not burn as they will.

Observation of the nuances of how a smudge herb responds to a situation contributes insight into what is happening and what is (or is not) present. The herb speaks through its smoke, revealing something of what is going on in the subtle realms. Blowing on smudge overrides its inclinations and information. Sometimes when an herb won't light it is telling you that smudge is not needed, or that something else should be done first. Often, its hesitation is because the smudging procedure is being initiated in too hasty, routine, or uncentered a manner. Over and over, little piles of sage leaves teach me to slow down, come back to quiet center, focus, ground myself, listen, be patient, be clear, and move from the heart with respect. Within the act of lighting the herb, then, is a chance to participate in spiritual awareness.

When you smudge someone, you move the smoke in a way that makes sense—you don't just waft it around. This is part of your clarity of purpose and procedure. You may choose a particular feather to help you, invoking that bird's medicine into partnership with the smudge herb. You may notice certain areas in the person's aura or body that call for extra attention, or you may guide the smoke more systematically, in whatever direction or sequence of movements seems fitting.

Quick smudges are analogous to splashing water on hands and face, while thorough, patiently delivered smudges are like long showers. Afterward you feel refreshed, relaxed, and focused. People skilled at smudging have a medicine gift.

Daily smudging is useful in conjunction with ceremony; illness or injury; emotional trauma; nightmare; mental preoccupation; depression; initiation of new projects, dwellings, relationships, and journeys; clearing and maintenance of medicine objects; and creation and protection of inviolate spaces.

I am staying the winter in an old farmhouse. It is too big for the three of us—several upstairs rooms are unused and the house feels haunted by previous occupants. I hear odd noises at night and catch glimpses of moving shapes. I mention this unpleasantness to the medicine man who is my mentor and he offers to carry out a house clearing. One afternoon I come home to find a braid of sweetgrass wreathed around my doorknob with a note attached to it. The medicine man found no one home, so he left the sweetgrass to use in clearing the house myself.

After lighting the end of the braid, I go from room to room spreading smoke into every corner, praying aloud. As I proceed I become more and more assertive, reclaiming the empty rooms, the damp cellar, the dark closets, occupying them with a firm presence that is reiterated, in Beauty, by the sweet smoke of the herb.

The process of clearing or smudging can help you realize the basis of fears and transform them to a basis of spiritual strength. That transformation is as much part of clearing as the actual effect of the plant. As with shamanic healing with herbs, you seek alignment with the plant's vision of wellness. You have the opportunity to welcome accord with whatever sacred truth is embodied by the herb. The subtle, pervasive nature of smoke, the transformative presence of fire, and the evocative medicine of the plant's fragrance release the herb's essential message into deep levels of consciousness. Those are mirrored in the unseen realms. Clarity in causative levels echoes to manifestive planes; integration flows in both directions.

Smudging strengthens reality because it is something you do, not just something you ponder or believe in. It is an active association of substance with essence. Smudging suggests that clarity is possible—it assumes a primary reality of well-being and integrity.

A woman brings two drums she and her husband used during their involvement with a shamanistic drumming group. She feels that the group's leader is manipulative and has gone astray into dark practices. She and her husband have withdrawn from the group but feel that, despite efforts at clearing, the drums somehow allow a link between them and the manipulative group leader. The woman wants me to have the drums, though I tell her I will almost certainly pass them on to someone else after clearing them. She decides that whatever I do with them is acceptable to her.

On examination, I find the drums not particularly affected by the group leader's influence but laden with the confusion, disillusionment, and fears of the woman and her husband. It is difficult to clear something if its undesirable charge is a reflection of your own emotions. The woman is wise to ask for help, but clearing the drums is not the solution to her and her husband's distress, nor will it break the unhappy link between them and the group leader.

I smudge the drums with sage and sweetgrass, and also clear them with light, water, and obsidian. It is a simple procedure—the drums' truths of being are easily acknowledged and restored. I pray during the clearing process. Afterward, I wrap the drums and store them in a closet. If in a year the woman moves to greater clarity, it will be time to return the drums; otherwise, they will be sent elsewhere.

Smudge herbs, like offering herbs, are teachers about how to live in good relationship with the larger community of life. They remind us to tend to the less visible aspects of presence and interaction. They remind us of the difference between looking neat and being clean. They give us a way to take action and to reach across the realms. The herb's giveaway into the fire quietly offers us the opportunity to let go and begin again.

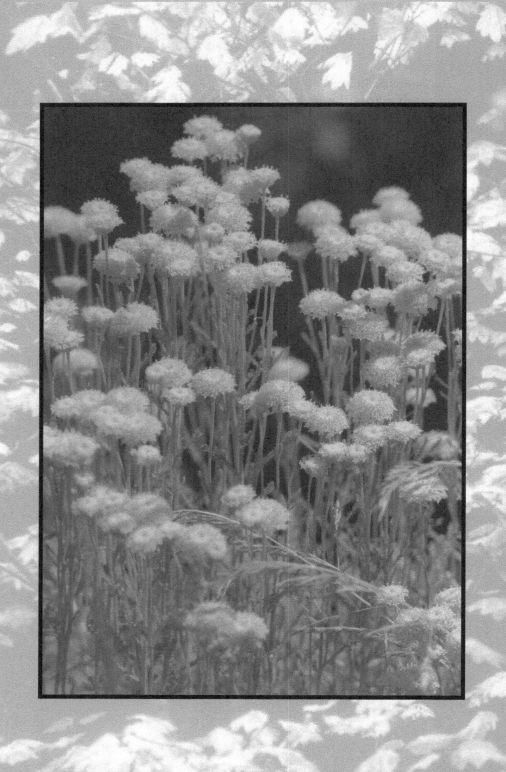

Chapter 7

Maintenance Herbs

It is our first spring equinox on the mountain. Since Imbolc there have been two pouches on the altar, both containing stones, crystals, and herbs. On equinox I give one pouch to my land partner and I take the other.

My land partner goes with her daughter to the southeast and southwest corners of the land we live on, and my son and I take our pouch to the northeast and northwest corners. The pouch's contents are divided and buried at those places. My son and I sit cupping the herbs and stones in our hands; we listen to the birds, the frogs, the wind; we watch a hawk wheeling above, a buttercup nodding in the breeze. Each good thing we see, hear, smell, and feel becomes part of the prayer with which we bury the herbs and stones. All those living things are the blessings—the beauty that makes land and life sacred to us. In our prayer we invoke protection, the strength of the sacred to endure. We entwine our lives with the truth of the mountain, asking and offering sanctuary. The herbs and stones keep watch, and remind us of our commitment.

When it is time to build our house, we construct footings for the foundation. Before cement is poured along the foundation's perimeter, I sprinkle crystals, tobacco, sage, rose petals, corn kernels, bits of cedar foliage, and sweetgrass into the footings, making prayers as I do so. Later, on the centerpost of the house, I hang feathers in the four directions, and pouches containing herbs and stones. I feel a sense of concentric extension emanating from the herbs and stones on the centerpost, in the foundation perimeter, and at the corners of our pact with the land.

Herbs can help delineate and maintain integrity of space. Dried herbs can be buried, strewn, or placed in containers, alone or with companion stones and crystals. Live plants can be cultivated in the ground or in pots. Cactus is a good guardian plant, indoors or out, as are other prickly "warrior" plants.

Protective herbs establish a presence that transmutes or wards off negativity. Alliance with those plants teaches and reminds you to dwell in your own light of being in such a way as to provide no resonant entrance for ill or fear of ill. The plants are not so much barriers as affirmations of good. Their attributes, whether of courage, strength, clarity of identity, guardianship, purity, or transformative power, assert a positive perspective. Allied with that view, you support integrity rather than defend against adversity. Once again, you align yourself with a vision of wellness, rejoining a reality of intrinsic wholeness.

Herbs are often placed in sacred bundles or with medicine objects to maintain the object's clarity of energy. Prairie sage and sweetgrass are frequently chosen for this. It is wise to periodically replace herbs being used for protection: burning or burying the plant material with prayers of gratitude. Highly charged articles, such as talons, claws, and ceremonial weapons, are partnered with protective herbs not only for the guardianship of the objects but for responsible containment of their predatory energies.

Less volatile objects can be well maintained through companionship with such herbs as rose petals, lavender, cedar, star anise, calendula, white sage, hyssop, and orris root. Crystals and stones, totem objects, and other ceremonial tools benefit from storage, or periodic renewing, in wrappings or in boxes, baskets, or pouches filled with herbs. Corn pollen or tobacco can be offered as nourishment for those objects. I often include a piece of obsidian in wrappings or containers housing medicine objects.

Like those employed for protection, herbs used for maintenance and renewal should also be rejuvenated or replaced from time to time. Looking at and handling those herbs informs you of when that needs to be done, or you can synchronize your rotations with moon phases or other natural cycles. Herbs that look and smell fresh and vibrant will be most effective.

I put maintenance and protection herbs in my vehicle and on my person as well as in my household. I use them in travel bundles, during legal matters, and in relation to the safety of my son and other loved ones. Like smudging, the use of maintenance and protective herbs requires attentiveness to subtle presences and movements, and includes those subtle levels of awareness in daily consciousness. It encourages proper respect and care for medicine objects and for the spaces around you. Draping a braid of sweetgrass over my mirror frame both reminds me to smudge myself and to see myself as a blessed and sacred being. I sometimes put small braids of sweetgrass on top of picture frames holding photographs of family, friends, or students. Sweetgrass can be laid beside or under the pillow of anyone troubled by nightmares or intrusive, nonordinary presences in her room during sleep.

Maintenance and protection herbs can also be applied in the form of essential oils, massage oils, bath herbs, or vapor herbs. Objects, people, or spaces can be anointed, washed, or suffused with herbal essences.

On the surface, much of herbal magic and folklore may appear superstitious, childish, or arbitrary, but through open-minded inquiry into the nature of plants you find that there is a sensible and enduring basis for magical herbalism. Like any system, it can be engaged and understood on many levels. Just as a nursery rhyme can be an allegory to the initiated, so a "lucky herb" can be a profound teacher to someone seeking deeper insight into herbs. The Druids, healers, magicians, and shamans of old were not fools. Their relationship with plants and trees has much to demonstrate to modern sophisticates about how to participate wisely in life's complex web.

Garden sage, for instance, is associated with wisdom and longevity. If you look within its virtues, you will find that sage has attributes very useful for menopausal women (wise women), and for elders in general. It is calming, antiseptic, astringent, antioxidant, keeps blood vessels and joints flexible, strengthens digestion and memory, and slows bodily aging. In traditional cultures, elders were valued and their experiences respected; thus, sage is linked with healthy, wise elders. Its medicine, like all herbs, speaks both physically and metaphysically. European herbal magic is grounded in practical knowledge.

Herbs can be used to invoke energies as well as maintain them. Incense is a form often chosen for creating specific vibrational atmospheres, and is used by many cultures. Smudging, as discussed in the preceding chapter, is one aspect of that use. Incense can catalyze shifts into meditative or altered states, especially if repeatedly used for that purpose. The incense fragrance, once familiar in attendance with a specific state, tends to induce that state more and more easily. This is not as effective if a fragrance is broadly used in association with a variety of activities and states of consciousness.

You may work with sun-loving plants for daytime incense use and nightblooming flowers for dream work, for example, or choose a traditional Eastern incense for meditation and use something indigenous for attuning to the local habitat.

Some incenses invoke spiritual presence better than others—some plants orient to specific deity forms and some to general vibrational states. It helps to check into traditional lore as well as to communicate with the plants you are interested in working with as invocational catalysts. Some plants, like frankincense and myrrh, blend well in partnership.

The same considerations apply to herbs used in the form of essential oils. Oils can be rubbed on candles or lightly applied to the body or clothing to make their fragrances available. Oils can be judiciously applied to appropriate chakra points, also, or chakra meditations can be supported by the burning of corresponding incenses.

Sometimes incense is used to bring calm or focus in a disturbed household or to unify a group embarking on a cooperative endeavor. Cultivating aromatic plants and flowering trees around or in your home is another way to invoke certain vibrational conditions.

I remember how, in early spring, the forest in northern Michigan smelled first of wild leeks, then of catnip. Where I live now, May is saturated with the heavenly fragrance of wild roses. Whether encountered spontaneously or through intention, scent is an evocative stimulant to consciousness. I once attended an eighteen-hour Native American Church ceremony during which great quantities of cedar were burned. For years afterward the smell of smoldering cedar sharply recalled the nausea so graphic in my memory of that experience. It took a long time for cedar smudge to once again evoke a wider range of ceremonial association.

Herbs for protection, maintenance, and invocation are hardworking allies integrated into the foundations of daily spiritual practice. Like the herbs in the footings of my house, they can set or sustain a tone of relationship with the larger matrix.

There are certain plants and trees of protection that, throughout my life, have appeared unexpectedly and with great power at times or in places when I had need of blessing and assurance. The connectedness that blossoms through such experiences brings with it the gift of at-home-ness on Earth—the trust that loving resource embodies itself throughout life.

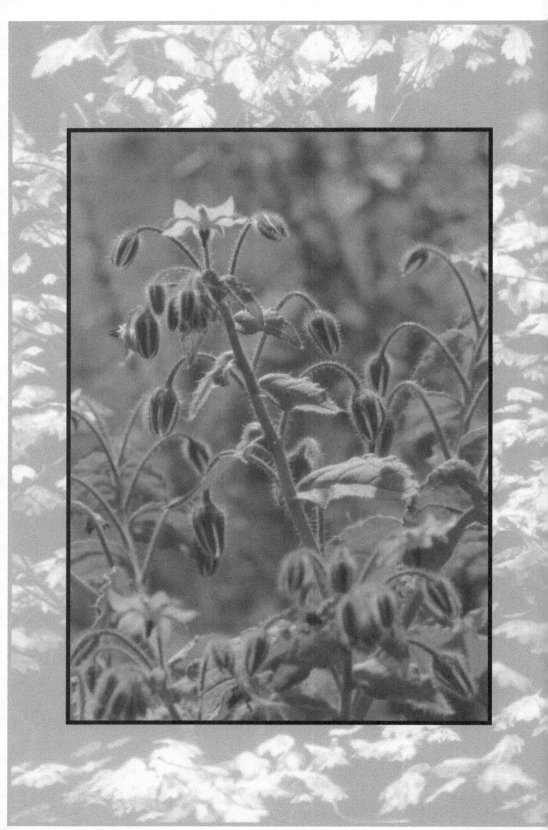

Chapter 8

Ceremonial Herbs

Just as shamans in modern times have access to a planetary cornucopia of herbs, so is a global array (or disarray) of ceremonial forms available to contemporary practitioners. Eclecticism is a sign of the times, for better or worse. Within sight of where I sit grow naturalized knapweed, mullein, yarrow, St. Johnswort, cinquefoil, and many other nonindigenous wild plants. Their ancestors, like mine, did not originate on this land, but here we are, now part of this habitat. Migrations of plants, people, and other beings constantly change the face of the Earth, change balances, change cultures. Movement is part of life, though some things stay in one place longer than others.

When engaging in ceremony, it is useful to consider the roots of what you do; the depth of your knowledge, skill, and attunement; and the larger resonances within culture and community. The use of herbs in ceremony is not separate from those considerations.

Unless you are trying to replicate a nonlocal, established ritual, it makes sense to ceremonialize with plants that grow locally. Historically, ceremony arose from and was intrinsic to its immediate habitat. The herbs involved were relevant to the situation, needs, and pattern of life at hand. Ceremony expressed relationship with the land and its spiritual forces.

There is little purpose in ceremonially working with herbs

with which you have no relationship, or with herbs that have only distant connection to your habitat. Though each plant is unique, most have correlates, so you can usually find appropriate local counterparts for herbs that grow in other lands. Honoring the plants close to you opens the way for deeper engagement with your own habitat. This is a vital aspect of healthful community participation.

You tend to be directly concerned with proper harvest, identification, and handling of herbs when you use local plants. This benefits both the plant community and the ceremonial occasions of their use. If you are trying to connect with or include a faraway locale in ceremony, it is helpful to use plant material from that place; otherwise, local herbs may best express your immediacy of ceremonial purpose.

Traditional ceremony, in its natural cultural and environmental context, is intimate with the land that shaped it. The plants, objects, movements, regalia, pace, and very intentions of ceremony are derived from and reflect matters of habitat. If shamanism has a cross-cultural core, it also has an equally important diversity of manifestation invoked by details of local environment and cultural patterning.

Modern spiritual seekers sometimes subject herbs (and other things) to egoic inspection and judgment rather than inquiring of the larger web about what choices best serve the good of all. People declare, "I'm most comfortable using this herb" or "I like how these flowers enhance my ceremonial outfit" or "This plant connotes power, so I'll use it," and so on. As awareness matures, this kind of superficial attitude may shift into a humble equanimity that listens to Spirit's quiet recommendations. Self-knowing then takes on a wider meaning.

All the plants used in North America as smudge or offering herbs are also found in ceremonial roles. Those plants, and others, are integral participants in indigenous ceremonies. For instance, at a Plains Sun Dance you will likely see sage covering the ground in the sweat lodges and being rubbed on the bodies of those who sweat. Sage may also cushion the places where medicine pipes rest on the Earth, and be wreathed around the heads, ankles, and wrists of the dancers, as well as being burned as a smudge.

The sacred arbors may be thatched with cedar boughs. The teepee poles may be pine, and the sweat lodge frames willow. You will see sweetgrass tucked into medicine bundles and burned for blessing. Cottonwood or other trees form the bodies of drums. The Sun Dance itself centers around a ceremonial tree. Tobacco is used in prayer ties and in pipes, the stems of which are usually wooden. Plants are, of course, part of the celebratory feast, and supply fuel for campfires.

European shamanic ceremony is plant-filled also, epitomized in the herbcraft of Wicca and the tree-centered rituals of the Druids. The closer you look, the more aware you become of how large a part plants play in ceremonial as well as mundane life.

Ceremonial, shamanic, or magical application of herbs is useful to study, even if your primary engagement with plants is medicinal. Understanding a plant through its characteristic nature makes its properties easier to remember, gives greater depth to your knowledge, and promotes a more personal, lively relationship with the plant.

Consider myrrh (Commiphora myrrha), for example. In magic work, myrrh is associated with the moon and water, and with the Egyptian deity Isis. It is burned as a purifying incense to invoke peace and aid meditation, usually in partnership with frankincense. Myrrh is often part of funerals and of winter ceremonies, and is sometimes used for exorcism or clearing. How can knowing those things help you understand and remember myrrh's medicinal qualities? Remedially, myrrh is an excellent antiseptic (exorcism). As an astringent, it affects fluidity, as does the moon. Astringency is contractive—in winter we draw inward; in death we withdraw entirely. Myrrh is used as a gargle to tighten and disinfect (purify) sore gums, to alleviate bad breath (exorcism again), and as a powder to heal ulcerations (peace-bringing). It is simple to correlate its magical reputation with its medicinal uses. Knowing one aspect, whether the shamanic or the scientific, reinforces your recall of the other. This can be done with any plant.

As you become familiar with a plant's spiritual nature and the qualities of its personality, you begin to discern its specific healing powers. Traditional correspondences encode clues to this through references to astrology, deity forms, elements, and other associations. The esoteric language of magic and shamanism tends to be more evocative than is the vocabulary of science or modern herbalism. Those languages reflect differing perspectives but not divergent knowledge.

A ceremony is generally a reverent occasion, or at least one that takes you out of ordinary circumstances and mind-sets. When you use herbs in ceremony you are urged by the formality of the context to perceive and handle the herbs with reverence. This teaches right relationship. Without these formal occasions, it is easy to fall into thoughtless behaviors toward plants. Ceremony reawakens awareness and renews spiritual perspective. It is a reminder that plants are sacred beings whom you rely on in countless ways.

Ceremony can be specifically for or about plants. The yearly round of seasons provides a ceremonial cycle tuned to the rhythms of plants and the honoring of fruitful interaction. In my life the ceremonial cycle is expressed with varying degrees of formality and in many spontaneous ways.

My observation of this begins on my birthday—midwinter, on Candlemas (Imbolc). The increasing day-length inspires garden planning and the procuring of seeds. It is an initiatory time, a time when I feel awareness drawn below the surface of manifestation to where new life is gestating. I often do a sweat lodge as renewal for the coming cycle, rededicating myself to Spirit's guidance. Imbolc is also when I hang some of last year's sunflower seedheads on trees for the birds and put the rest on the ground for the animals. If I have dried ceremonial corn I put that out too, with gratitude that I have something to share from Earth's bountiful giveaway.

As leaf buds begin to swell at spring equinox, the midpoint between light and dark, I honor the trees in their beauty of balance between Earth and Sky. Sometimes I visit trees that I feel a particular affection for, communing with them, tying ribbons or offerings in their branches, wishing them well in the coming growing season. Between equinox and Beltane as the weather softens, I begin planting early vegetables in the garden. Before planting I converse with the spirits of the land and give tobacco offerings of thanks for the chance to live as I do and be fed from the garden.

At the beginning of May is Beltane, a time for rejoicing in the flowers, for celebrating aliveness, creativity, and beauty. The mountain I live on is at its softest now—barefoot time—before the heat and dryness of summer. I take walks and luxuriate in deep breaths of fragrant air. I praise the mosses, admire blossoms, caress leaves, and make love with the elements. I feel the mountain open itself to the season's embrace. In May I gather wild roses, welcome the sage harvest, and make fresh echinacea tincture.

Midsummer's eve is another time when I turn to the sweat lodge and to prayers burned in tobacco ties. Solstice is my favorite herb-gathering time, a time for gathering leaves and flowers, especially when solstice coincides with a full moon. The garden is fully planted. The long length of day allows me to gather wild herbs late into the evening, hands and leaves sunwarmed, blessed by an abundance of light. The tinctures and teas made from solstice herbs will bring summer's warmth and fullness of life into the winter ahead.

The creek's flow is small, the land dry and yet fruitful in August. At Lughnasad I pray for the serving of balances—for the land and the people. I pray to know what needs to be given and how best to participate in the web of life. I honor the springs and streams on the mountain and the food plants in the garden. After Lughnasad, there is a feeling of season's turning, the light lessening; in mid-August the trees begin hinting of autumn. I feel the moonlight ripening the grain.

Soon it is the time of the autumn equinox. Again the year pauses in balance. It is my land partner's birthday, and both her daughter and my son also have birthdays near equinox, so it is a celebratory time here. Autumn is a busy season, the momentum sweeping me toward winter. The pause at equinox is welcomed: an opportunity to take stock, center and clear, realign priorities, discern what to store and what to release. It is firewood-gathering time, and with deep gratitude I cut, haul, and stack what will enable me to survive on the mountain through winter. As at spring equinox, focus is drawn to the trees, beautiful now in their brilliant, dying leaves. The equinox feast honors harvest; between equinox and Samhain I put the garden to rest.

Samhain and Yule are often the most formal of the seasonally oriented ceremonies I celebrate. On Samhain eve is the feast for the dead, a silent ceremony and a time for remembering ancestors and loved ones who have passed. I do my final herb gathering before Hallows, digging roots to dry or tincture. Samhain eve is a good occasion for divination. One year I put the hollowed Samhain pumpkin outside after the ceremony, and a mouse moved into it for the winter.

The Yule log is part of my winter solstice ceremony: during our cold winters there is special appreciation for the trees who radiate their memories of heat and light within the woodstove's fire. Solstice is a magically charged time for me with its crystalline silence—peaceful conception in the depth of night. My son and I hang fir and pine boughs around our big picture window and dangle ornaments from them. The boughs we cut with prayer and companionableness, and on solstice we breathe the silence and the dark, then light candles and sing.

It is interesting to consider how meaningful it is—how validating of spiritual experience —when significant physical manifestations occur during ceremony. When, for example, an affirmative charge is felt when you lift your arms to the sky in prayer, and an eagle glides past. For all the discounting of physicality that is heard in the metaphysical community, there is still a great importance placed on material reinforcement of spiritual experience. This is good, not because materiality is a measure of spirit's presence and power, but because it is vital that sacredness not dwell in a realm apart from earthly life. Ceremony needs to be firmly connected to physical experience so that we develop an integral awareness and interact with what is around us in a sacred way.

I include a Yule log in my solstice ceremony, not because it is an ancestral tradition, but because the hearth is the core of my survival in winter. It is where I burn trees in order to heat food, water, and my home. To be in good relationship with those trees, I feel a need to ceremonially honor them, and to carry that awareness and gratitude into daily manifestation through right relationship with the trees. The explicit realization of interdependency gives ceremony greater power and meaning.

It is early spring on the mountain, the leaves not yet unfurled, and I go to my medicine wheel to make prayers. There is never much vegetation on the rocky outcrop the wheel rests upon, where the mountain's bones show through the thin, dry soil.

I step to the stone marking East and make my prayer. When I bend down to lay tobacco on the stone, I am arrested by the sight of a single flower blooming exactly in front of the marker, a buttercup holding the East's golden light. Gazing at its innocent perfection, I am reminded again that life, itself, is the magic.

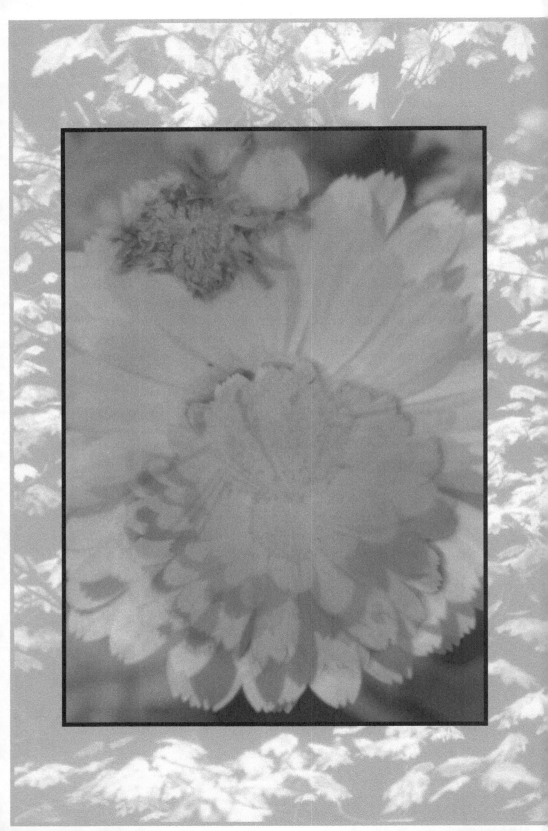

Chapter 9

Smoking Herbs and Use of Psychotropic Plants

Tobacco was referred to in the chapter on herbal offerings, and in discussing ceremonial plants. Though many herbs can be smoked, tobacco is usually the first plant that comes to mind when smoking is mentioned, with marijuana a close second.

Breath is a vehicle of the sacred, and a vehicle of life itself. Breath is the focus of meditation and the carrier of prayer, song, and chant. It is a gift renewed moment by moment until death, a constant cycle of embrace and release. To merge the breath with smoke from a burning plant is to invite an intimacy of essence with essence. When used in ceremony, smoking is the breath made visible: prayer made visible, intention joined with substance, mingling with the airs that are shared by all. Air is used in common—no one has a private stock. What is put into the air, whether words, sounds, smells, or smoke, should ideally express respect for the gift of breath and the commonality of air. As I used to say to my son when he experimented with silly noises: "That sound will forever remain in the universe."

The ceremony of smoking proceeds in acute awareness of what is being released into the universe. The focus is on truth, gratitude, and harmonious relationship. When the same plants and the same ritual actions used by someone for ceremony are also used in careless or abusive ways, it may be worthwhile for the person to reexamine his or her spiritual alignment with the smoking herb and smoking as a ceremonial act.

Using an herb as a sacrament is tricky business. Most if not all herbs used sacramentally, whether smoked or ingested, have strong psychoactive natures or are easily habit-forming or toxic. Traditionally they were used by spiritual specialists who understood the natures of the plants—and their own natures— and who followed ceremonial protocols indicating when and how the plants were approached.

What can be observed in much of contemporary sacramental use of herbs is a spiritual veneer covering desires or needs that are not congruent with sacred purpose. The nature of those herbs willingly obliges subjective illusion, making it all the more difficult for people to clearly perceive their true pattern of relationship with the herb.

I have noticed that practitioners who use powerful herbs (other than tobacco) sacramentally also tend to engage in casually habitual use of other "drug" plants and energy modifiers. If you are attracted to plants such as marijuana, peyote, psilocybin, and so on, you may want to seek perspective about what it is in you that wants or finds resonance with those beings. When working with them, by all means treat them sacramentally, but beware of self-delusion. With smoking herbs, greater clarity may be found in using ceremony itself, rather than psychoactive plants, as the sacrament.

It is Imbolc and I am attending an open community celebration. As we sit around the campfire, a man loads a large ceremonial pipe and hands it to me; I assume he does this because I am often asked by the community to lead ceremonies. I light the pipe and quietly pray with it, smoking all its contents and handing it back to its owner. The man, a consternated look on his face, hurriedly puts the pipe away, looking subdued. My husband, sitting beside me, tries to look subdued also, but is almost tearful from suppressed laughter.

"What's so funny?" I ask him.

"The pipe," he chortles. "You just smoked a pipeload of pot—didn't you notice? He obviously intended to impress people by passing it around the crowd. You single-handedly turned his expensive pipeful into ashes."

Oriented to prayerful intent, and buffered by innocence, despite my past experience with marijuana, I had no realization that the herb I was smoking was marijuana, and received no drug effect from smoking it.

It is worthwhile to consider what is being shared when people come together seeking attunement. Smoking marijuana is a tradition of my generation's counterculture and is still connected to ideals of liberty and communalness, as well as to nostalgia for the days when we were young and felt revolutionary. Under that haze of communal smoke, however, abided sexism, factionalism, racial tensions, shortsightedness, egotism, and pain. Marijuana was a common bond, a common language of lifestyle, but not a healer of our common suffering.

Many people of my generation still use marijuana to relax, and to create a sense of group sociability and solidarity in conjunction with both mundane and ceremonial occasions. Smoking is a ritualistic process, becoming even more ritualistic when done in a group. The intimate passing of a joint or pipe from hand to hand/mouth to mouth/breath to breath weaves its particular spell.

This ritual is entangled with the suffering within prevalent patterns of relationship and self-perception. There is an observable difference in how people in a traditional pipe ceremony respond to someone who does not smoke—who touches the pipe to brow or heart instead of inhaling—and in how people sharing a joint respond to someone who does not partake. In the first situation there is no division or disattunement; in the second, there usually is, even if subtle. Most people who quit smoking marijuana find that quitting affects how their friends who continue to smoke interact with them.

If feelings of inclusion and mutuality depend on an external agent, then whatever is being shared or attuned to is not intrinsic spiritual alignment. If feelings of connection only last as long as the agent's effects, then its use is not fostering actual or enduring trust, acceptance, or congeniality.

Why are the powerful experiences of sweat lodge, ecstatic dance, lovemaking, shamanic drumming, and so on not sufficient in themselves to people who combine them with consciousness modifiers such as marijuana? Is there fear that the doors to mystery will not otherwise open or that sensations will not be extraordinary enough? Is there a need to try to enhance perception of primal energies? Are people at a loss for how to access attunement through the unaugmented vehicles of mind, body, spirit, and heart?

We arrive at the question of discernment between neediness and alliance. Ultimately, what can be realized is a transcendent perspective of wholeness and self. It is difficult to reach this when you tie yourself to assumptions of limitation. Alliance is not dependency: it is interdependency, an expanded experience of self. When you call on an ally's help, you do so not out of personal lack but out of recognition of larger self. There is a profound difference between the two, discernible in how people use consciousness-altering plants.

When a plant is used due to lack of vision, lack of attunment, lack of disciplined attention, lack of sociability, lack of fluid consciousness, lack of imagination, and so on, its use is resonant with inadequacy, not with spiritual reality. This appears, to subtle perception, as the would-be ally overshadowing or dominating an egoic consciousness. When invocation of an ally is resonant with wholeness or healthy relationship, it manifests as a clarity of undivided presence, spiritually aligned. Such invocation is not done to compensate for lack but to utilize or animate an aspect of wholeness. This can certainly apply to tobacco, marijuana, peyote, and other plant allies, but it requires self-honesty, wisdom, and healthy alignment.

For many people of my generation, psychotropic plants were

the doorway into experiences of expanded consciousness. Mind-altering drugs are generally a "break-and-enter" way of passing through that doorway, however, and can thereby contribute to outright damage or to formation of belief that expanded consciousness can only be reached through extreme measures or with the help of external agents. This consequence can create the illusion of a closed door, cause fear of that passage into expanded awareness, or generate a constellation of obstructive or problematic beliefs, doubts, and attachments concerning the use of psychotropic plants.

A less loaded arena to consider is the simple use of smoking herbs for prayer and healing. Many herbs lend themselves to this. Mullein and coltsfoot can be used as bases for smoking blends and as healers for throat and lung ailments. (Inhalation of any herb's smoke is detrimental if overdone.) Other respiratory herbs occasionally smoked are comfrey, plantain, horehound, and red sage. Coltsfoot and skullcap are smoked for asthma. Some herbs, like ginseng, dandelion, and cinquefoil, are stimulating smokes, and skullcap, catnip, passion flower, violet, wild lettuce, borage, chamomile, meadowsweet, and lavender are relaxing. (Wild lettuce is sedative; use with care.)

Uva ursi and red willow are often smoked in Native kinnikinnick blends. Datura (poisonous), damiana, muscadine, and wormwood are also smoked, but should be approached with caution, if at all. Spearmint is often added to blends to buffer the harsher smoke of some plants. Healing or prayer herbs can be smoked in pipes, rolled into cigarette papers or corn husks, or burned in shallow dishes or bowls.

Use of hallucinogenic plants is a controversial subject. There is a tendency for people to gravitate to one pole of opinion or the other, leaving the middle ground unexplored. I am neither for nor against their use. My thoughts are about how—not whether—people engage with particular plants. The following are some steps that might be taken in developing a good alliance with a plant such as peyote or one of the hallucinogenic mushrooms.

1. Consider the path that has brought you into encounter with the plant. Contemplate its implications and the influences surrounding it.
2. Learn about the plant's physicality and its historical usage. Talk to people who work with it. Read about it. If possible, observe it growing in its natural habitat.
3. Greet the plant's spirit and ask for knowledge and understanding of the plant. Continue until you can clearly hear and see the spirit (without ingesting the plant), and communicate with it. Ask how to be in good relationship with it.
4. Dream the plant. Sleep with it under your pillow. Seek its teachings in nonordinary states of consciousness. Ask for a song or prayer associated with it. Meditate on the plant. Put a photo or drawing of it on your altar, along with some of the wrapped plant material.
5. Carry the plant on your person. Become familiar with its presence. Hold it in your hands. Pray with it. Smudge it. Continue to deepen your communication and spiritual resonance. Call on its help, still without ingesting the plant's substance.
6. Set the plant aside in a respectful, grateful manner. Seek guidance from the Source. Seek perspective and wisdom. Examine your intentions, your shadows, your patterns, and your desires. Give time to this—perhaps a moon cycle.
7. If the path of alliance indicates this, reapproach the plant. Smudge it and yourself. Pray, addressing the plant's spirit with clear intention. Align yourself with Source and plant. Ingest its medicine in a sacred way.

Using those steps, or something similar, you move through a deepening unfoldment of relationship rather than immediately hopping into bed together (so to speak). The attunement may or may not consummate in physical union. That sort of movement facilitates respectful, knowledgeable, productive, and clear interaction with the plant, giving alliance a spiritual basis.

As I am dressing after a sweat lodge, I notice one of the participants hand something to another. It is too dark to discern the gift's form. What I see is prismatic light in the person's cupped hands, as though she holds a palmful of multicolored gleams. The gift is tucked away, the strong presence of its medicine muffled. I finish dressing. Later, the gift's receiver tells me that she had been given a handful of hallucinogenic mushrooms.

Those whose perceptions and responses are naturally sensitive or sensitized through practice may find it more beneficial to work with certain plant alliances through touch or visual focus rather than through ingestion. Shifting to that level of attunement bypasses physical concerns and reliances. It engages the plant on a level that exercises your capacity to access altered states using more subtle forms of induction.

Whether your expression of good relationship with a plant is to ingest it or to not ingest it, the choice should emerge from freedom of consciousness. Plants can open doors for you, but if what you carry through those thresholds is the baggage of fear, confusion, egoic desires, insecurity, and illness of relationship, your journey will be circumscribed by those burdens. Psychotropic plants are powerful teachers, guides, and medicine beings. They expand awareness but explicitly mirror alignment of consciousness.

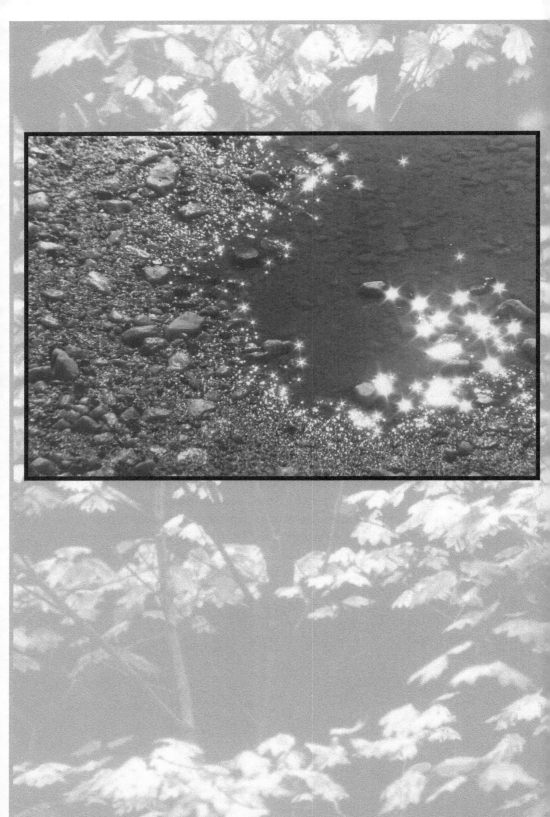

Chapter 10
Birth, Death, and Dreaming Herbs

Birth, death, and dreaming are events unto themselves, but their natures are transitional. The herbs that companion those events are initiatory, supportive, and complementary.

It is true that nothing in life is the same as birth, death, or dreaming, but much in life is compared to those experiences. They are metaphors for many other passages. Herbs that are traditional allies for birth, death, and dreaming are appropriately used in situations that involve similar energies.

Birth is an incarnational journey—acceptance of participation in a certain strata of experience. Birth is transformation's embodiment, the initiation of a new cycle. The energies surrounding birth, whether literal childbearing or metaphoric birth, could be seen as a cycle within a cycle, beginning with fertility.

Fertility exemplifies the ability to embark on birth's cycle. In a sacred sense, it implies not only willingness, but also capacity and wise timing, the allies of conception. Herbs that nourish fertility are fenugreek seeds, lemon balm, false unicorn root, red clover flowers, dong qui, red raspberry leaves, saw palmetto berries, squawvine, and black haw.

Conception bridges fertility and gestation. Gestation is a phase that begins in the hidden realm and gradually reveals itself in visible and substantial expression. Herbs of gestation are red raspberry leaves, ginger root, anise seeds, nettles, yellow dock root, dandelion leaves, oatstraw, and alfalfa.

Gestation culminates in labor, an effort and surrender guided by the intelligence and power of natural process. Herbs that can help you labor include blue and black cohosh, ginger root, cotton root bark, spikenard, skullcap, and raspberry leaves. Sometimes the emergence in birth can shift to emergency, and plants that aid in times of such difficulty are angelica root, blue cohosh, shepherd's purse, ground ivy, motherwort, evening primrose, lobelia, lady's mantle, and witch hazel.

Birth is the cycle's climax but not its end. Postpartum involves integration, nurturance, and devolution. Herbs that partner this phase are fennel seeds, blessed thistle, borage, hops, lemon balm, motherwort, and (again) red raspberry leaves. The birth cycle can be likened to the moon's: new moon is fertile, waxing moon is gestational, full moon is labor's culmination, and waning moon is similar to the postpartum period.

I have purposely not described how or under what physical circumstances to apply birth herbs. The use of plants in childbearing is a field of study in itself. What is indicated in this brief overview is the correlation between certain herbs and the energies of birth's cycle. The details a childbirth practitioner or birthing mother needs to know go beyond this in order to make use of it in practice. Using these herbs to accompany metaphoric birth or similar processes is not so exacting an application.

For example, to bring a project to fruition you might prepare for its inception by drinking lemon balm or fenugreek tea as you sit contemplating your ideas. Once your plans start to materialize, you might make and carry an amulet of gestational herbs, or surround a written description of your project with such herbs. As the project reaches fulfillment you might shift to an amulet of labor herbs, use labor herbs as prayer offerings, or nourish yourself with raspberry leaf tea. If the project is beset by difficulties you might burn angelica incense, or ask for spiritual help from birth's other emergency herbal allies. During the project's postpartum phase you might wind down with infusions of fennel, lemon balm, or borage, or take a bath with hops flowers, or use blessed thistle as an offering herb of gratitude and completion.

The physiologic process of birth contains interesting paradoxes that can be considered during situations mirroring birth. The uterus contracts so that the cervix can open; after birth, stimulation to the breasts causing milk to flow also causes the womb to clamp down, constricting blood vessels at the placental site; labor's work requires relaxed surrender, but also endurance, strength, and determination; birth is a letting go that allows arrival, and it is an organic process that encompasses metaphysical, transcendent experience.

Herbs that are allies to birth are contractive or astringent (saw palmetto, squawvine, black haw, blue cohosh, cotton root, shepherd's purse, and witch hazel, for instance), or expansive and fluid-producing (anise seeds, oatstraw, motherwort, and borage, for example). As a group they teach a wisdom of right timing: when to push, when to sit back; when to gather and focus resources and when to disperse them. The medicine of those herbs is about pace, rhythm, and effort in harmony with natural unfoldment.

Red raspberry is the plant most allied with birth's physical manifestation. The herb most linked with subtle energies of birth is lavender. Lavender has appeared to me during births as a blue-robed woman standing beside the bed. Rooms used for childbirth are sometimes washed with lavender infusion before labor begins, or the flowers are hung in doorways and over the bed. Lavender is a peace-bringer, its energy very calming and clearing. The fragrance of lavender is clean and soothing. The flowers are used medicinally as an antiseptic or to relieve headaches. They promote strength in the immune system, and can be infused into massage oil for rubbing on pregnant bellies. Lavender is a quiet guardian, but not a faltering one. Many midwives carry lavender in their birth kits, and revere her presence at births.

As birth is the time of first breath, so death is the moment of final breath. The passage from bodily to spiritual realm is a process of demanifestation. Having been midwife during both birth and death, I have seen their similarities and the ways in which they are opposite, though much of what polarizes them is the common response of rejoicing at one and grieving at the other.

Both birth and death have, unfortunately, been relegated mainly to hospital settings in modern times, thus turning them into medical events instead of natural passages. This has affected the experiences of being born and dying, and of witnessing those profound transitions. When such intimate moments are taken out of the hands of family, partners, and community, there is a great loss within humanity's shared experience. When birth and death are hidden away, surrounded by technology and severed from a continuity of loving, respectful interdependency, they become fearful, alien events.

Learning to take care of each other during birth and death is a large part of how mutual well-being is understood and expressed. A woman once said, "If all men attended the natural birthings of their children, there would be no more war." Being supportively present during those passages in and out of life makes life's sacredness more deeply realized.

Birth and death are everyday occurrences and are often messy, nitty-gritty affairs, yet even so there is an enduring sense of mystery surrounding them, a crossing into and out of the unknown. The plants associated with death both guard that mystery's threshold, giving comfort to those bereaved, and aid the journeying soul who passes beyond.

Periwinkles and violets are put on graves and coffins of children. Marjoram, star anise, parsley, bluebells, asphodel, willow, and aconite are grown on burial sites of adults. Aconite, basil, star anise, and myrrh are funeral incenses. Lotus and anemone are associated with favorable reincarnation.

In Europe, the body of the deceased was traditionally washed with asphodel, pennyroyal, or tansy infusion; rose petal or other flower washes honor the beauty of embodiment's blossoming and fading. Chervil or thyme can be ingested for communion with those who have passed, and European mandrake can be buried with the deceased as protection during the spirit's journey.

Herbs for dying invite courage and offer relief from pain. Some of them, like basil and aconite, are initiatory—herbs of transformation. Morphine is the plant derivative used medically for deliverance from pain and, sometimes, to ease passage into death.

Our friend, a young man of twenty-nine, releases his final breath at home, in the calm presence of loved ones. Some minutes after death, the room empties of people except for myself and the man's wife. We uncover his naked body and smudge it with sage and sweetgrass, then tenderly wash it with cooled rose petal infusion. The room is peaceful and quiet; a feeling of the man's spirit is still present.

I ceremonially cut the spirit's connection to the body with an abalone knife, talking to the man as I do so, speaking of his journey beyond this world. I put corn pollen on his eyelids, in his mouth, and on the palms of his hands, also touching his brow with the golden powder.

We wrap the body in a blanket, face uncovered, and tuck sage, sweetgrass, cedar, lavender, and other herbs within the blanket's folds. I make a prayer as candles and incense are lit; they will burn continuously beside the body until it is taken for cremation the following day. I say good-bye to my friend.

Like birth, death is a metaphor for other (nonlethal) experiences. Many crone rituals are death analogs. They focus on dissolution of substance or form—on destructuralization, transformation, transcendence, or release. In order for something to change or be renewed there must be death on some level. Winter precedes spring; night gives truth to dawn.

Mushrooms are associated with death and transformation. I am sometimes given teachings about mushrooms during my dreams. Shade-loving or night-blooming plants are allies of dreaming, death, and change, as are plants like willow that grow in or near water. Communion with those plants during the death phase of a transformational cycle may help you move with greater power as well as acceptance. Plants participate ungrudgingly in change—it is native to their medicine.

Many shamanic practitioners are attracted to toxic or perilous plants. Wolfbane (aconite), henbane, Mexican datura, morning glory, belladonna, opium poppy, and so on, have auras of risky power. They dangle the lure of alterations in consciousness and sensation. They grow on death's borderland. There is a fine line between easing pain and courting death, whether physical or metaphysical. It takes clarity to discern that line, and clarity to know if and when to cross it.

Passages, thresholds, and nonordinary terrains are shamanic precincts of practice—it is natural for dangerous, mysterious herbs to beckon those who move between the worlds. As in alliance with psychotropic mushrooms, cacti, and so on, focus needs to be on right relationship, the path of spiritual alignment.

Bridging herbs of birth and herbs of death are plants whose medicines celebrate sexuality. The primal fire of sexuality vitalizes life's dance and burns within shamanic work that serves life's web. Sexuality is inextricably linked to conception and birth, and to death's release and transcendent union.

Most of the herbs associated with sexuality are aphrodisiacs or stimulants. They include cubeb berries, damiana, henna, kava-kava, orchid, mandrake, hibiscus, cumin, male fern, rose geranium, ginseng, and yohimbe. Those herbs, used in a sacred way rather than as drugs to boost potency or sex drive, concentrate awareness and energy in the sexual fire. They are not herbs of temperance. If you tend to reach for outside modifiers to pace your energy through daily ups and downs, you may have cause to question your motives in using those plants.

Aphrodisiac herbs are, on the whole, warming and quickening. Some, like orchids, bear erotic-looking blossoms or, like rose geraniums, have sweet, heavy perfumes. The roots of mandrake and ginseng have a male or phallic appearance. Hibis-

cus, cumin, yohimbe, and henna carry the sensuality of tropical or hot climate zones.

Yohimbe is specific for problems of decreased pelvic circulation, low sperm motility, and depressed testosterone levels,
but is useful for short-term periods only. Damiana helps impo-
tence caused by anxiety or intellectual distraction. Two other
herbs, Virginia snakeroot and cotton-root bark, are used simi-
larly; snakeroot to counteract emotional distraction and cotton
root to stimulate contractile tissues. These herbs are ones having a clearly medicinal affect on sexuality and potency.

When aphrodisiac or stimulant herbs are used in conjunction with lovemaking, magic, or medicine work, they should
be present as partners, not as forces that dominate, manipu-
late, or obscure spiritual intention and response. Any plant that
alters consciousness or has a radical effect on the body is will-
ing to magnify your shadows, if that is what, in essence, you
are asking of it. I once told my sweetheart that it bothered me
to have him make love to me when he was high on marijuana
because it was like having an uninvited third person in bed
with us. Additional partners should be present on such occasions only if all involved welcome it.

Dreams are another nonordinary terrain in which herbs offer
guidance, help, or companionship. The dream realm may be
where you most distinctly see, hear, or interact with certain allies,
or where teachings are given and shamanic work carried out.

To reach the dream realms, you first need to fall asleep. Herbs
can facilitate sleep or help create states conducive to vivid
dreaming. Those herbs are either smoked (catnip, damiana),
burned (mugwort, damiana, rosemary), taken as a tincture or
tea (mint, vervain, catnip, passion flower, lesser celandine), or
put into pillows that are placed near your head (meadowsweet,
betony, mugwort, rosemary, anise seeds, mimosa flowers, wisteria flowers, thyme, lavender, hops, lemon balm, lemongrass,
chamomile, hyssop, sweet woodruff, rose petals, scented geraniums, agrimony, purslane, mint, oakmoss, narcissus flowers,
cowslip, violet, hyacinth, tuberose).

By far, the herb most often used for strong dreaming is mugwort. This plant, like prairie sage and wormwood, is one of the Artemisias—associated with Artemis, protector and huntress of wild creatures and keyed to Artemis's lunar influences. As with most dream practices, you may need to use mugwort a number of times before perceiving results, though some people describe immediate, dramatic changes in their dream experiences when they begin working with mugwort.

Dream herbs awaken subtle levels of attention, soften barriers between waking and sleeping, or calm the mind. Some are romantic plants. The sleep herbs (catnip, chamomile, agrimony, passion flower, skullcap, vervain, valerian, hops, lavender, and wild lettuce) are remedial nervines or sedatives. Other night allies are guardians (rosemary, lavender, betony, anise, wild thyme, and hyssop), or align you with peace (purslane, costmary, lesser celandine, lemon balm, oakmoss, cowslip, and violet). Some encourage a state of receptivity (meadowsweet, mimosa, wisteria, lemongrass, sweet woodruff, rose petals, scented geraniums, narcissus, hyacinth, tuberose), and some are directly affiliated with dream states (damiana, mugwort).

One night when my son was a child, I heard him exclaim in his sleep. The house was still; the single word rang out in a tone of wonder and happiness: "Roses!" May we all dream so sweetly.

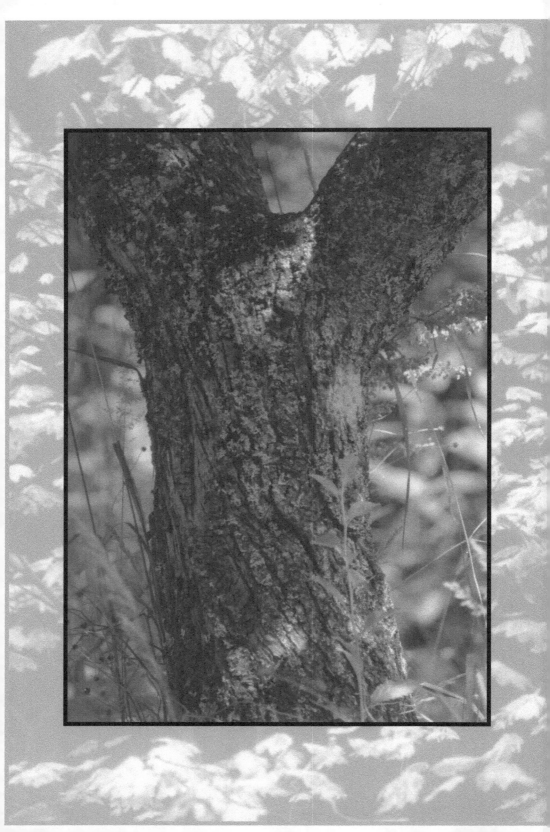

Chapter 11

Trees

The sun over the everglades is hot, as it is always hot. I stand on the raised boardwalk, gazing at the tree in front of me—the oldest mahogany left alive in the United States. It has pale gray, smooth bark over a muscular-looking trunk. I lean forward, over the boardwalk's railing, and rest my hand on the tree's skin.

The sodden heat, whining insects, long-legged birds, viperous snakes, and swampy waters of the everglades are not strange to me—I was born in Florida. The old tree and I have common roots. Tourist sandals clack on the board like the clicking shutters of busy cameras. The tree stands, patient in the broiling sunlight, the last of its age.

Sheep have grazed the gently rolling hills until their green cover is like a threadbare rug. My son and I stand in the shade of a thick-trunked, wide-canopied tree, reading the painted sign beside it. In the near distance rises the pink stone majesty of Drumlanrig castle. The tree is the largest remaining sycamore in Great Britain. We have wandered away from the castle and come upon this extraordinary tree.

The sign tells us that the trunk's girth is 6.6 meters—almost twenty-two feet around. Heavy branches slant outward beginning low on the trunk. My son finds a comfortable niche and rests, seated on the broad knee of one of the sycamore's roots. I pick up a winged seed, one of hundreds the tree has cast to the winds: its dreams and memories. Perhaps some will take root. I leave tobacco and a prayer, carrying that one seed home, a small but potent hope for the future.

Driving down the northern California coast, we arrive amid the thin corridor of the world's remaining redwoods. We get out of the car. My husband goes one way and I another. After all the oohing and ahhing together it is time for solitary contemplation.

The trees are beyond all familiar proportions, even for someone who lives beside the giant firs and cedars of the Olympic Peninsula. The redwoods are awesome, both in the ancient meaning of the word and in the original experience of awe. I lean my body, arms outspread, against one of those vast beings, my cheek resting on the deeply furrowed bark. Old. The tree has seen so much. My tears slide like salty coastal rain on the redwood's trunk. I cannot bear the thought of these trees cut. People in our society think computers are such a big deal, that technology is such a big deal. But they're not.

The chapters of this book unfolded like a cycle of seasons. They began with the springtime focus on gardening and gathering, gaining experience, and learning to prepare plants as remedies. The chapters proceeded to summerish concerns of relationship and alliance, and on to autumnal involvement with ceremonial and magical realms. Winter's energies emerged in the chapter on birth, death, and dreaming herbs and here, in this final chapter on the elders of the plant world. When I outlined the book I did not have that seasonal or medicine wheel configuration consciously in mind; it was as I began writing this chapter that the pattern became apparent. All the books I have written carry this pattern because it is a mandala of natural experience. Trees epitomize the teachings of seasonal cycles.

When my son was small he thought trees moved at night when no one was looking, and that the rustling of their leaves caused the movement of wind. He recognized trees as powerful beings. A logger who recently quit his job told his baffled, scornful supervisor that he was quitting because he could hear falling trees screaming in his sleep. When you take serious note of trees your sense of life changes.

For the shamanic herbalist, trees are allies that, like herbs, offer their vision in support of healing. Because they are long-lived, individual trees may become beloved presences who inspire, offer comfort, delight, and shelter you.

The web of communication among trees, in which humans can participate, operates through root systems, mycelium networks, and leaf activity. Trees growing near sacred wells or springs were traditionally venerated—the movement of underground water is another part of communication's web, and also a conduit for physical and spiritual nourishment.

In European pagan tradition, different species of trees were considered embodiments of or connections to various deities. Offerings, prayers, and petitions to deities were made directly to their tree embodiments. Some oft-visited trees became heavily bedecked with ribbons, coins, bits of colored cloth, jewels, and weapons. Wood henges or sacred groves were sites where Druids and pagans worshiped.

In Native shamanism, tree spirits were invited into carved masks, such as the ones used by the Iroquois False Face Society or some of the masks and carvings made by northwest coastal artists. The making of such vitalized masks is a meticulous process that involves knowledge of esoteric mysteries and spiritual intimacy with trees, as well as woodworking skills.

Trees killed for ceremonial use should be taken only at true need, and in a sacred manner that rests upon the tree's cooperation. Branches, foliage, or bark should be harvested with respect and gratitude. In today's world, where trees are becoming scarce and have been treated with brutality, greed, or indifference, it is important to look deeper into how much and in what way you use trees in your spiritual as well as your mundane affairs.

Out of consideration for the current situation, I try to have a light touch when cutting cedar boughs for a ceremony, or gathering birch bark for firestarter, or selecting saplings for a lodge. The trees can't afford our continued profligacy. It is time to reassess participation in the community of life, and to change consumptive habits.

I remember a ceremony I once attended with four hundred other people during which a silent standing meditation was done. We were asked to join hands in a huge circle and meditate on being trees. The ceremony took place in a grassy clearing surrounded by trees; at one point during the meditation I opened my eyes and it seemed that the people in the circle had truly become rooted, a grove within a grove. There was such peace and silence, just the breeze riffling our leaves and the summer sun stirring our cells, helping us grow. I have since used tree meditations with workshop students, and always there is that same quiet happiness, the balance between Earth and Sky.

My mother teaches the children in our rural, home-schooling community. I walk to her house from mine, hoping to have a word with her. As I approach the house I hear her voice. She is reading a story aloud to the children, but at first I can't see where she is. Then I smile—she is seated on a branch of the comfortable beech tree growing on the forest's verge, and perched on various other branches, like bright-eyed, bright-feathered birds, are the listening children.

PART 2
MATERIA MEDICA

Grace
in the seedhead
bending
August.
Grace in the
depths
of the forest
green-guarded.
Grace
in the hills
clothed in dreams
of home.
The light
upon the stones
keeps me.

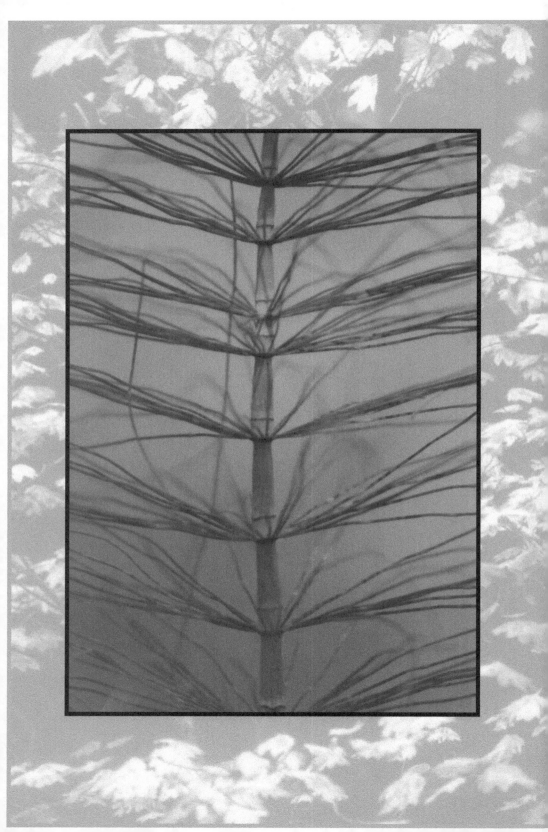

Rather than giving exhaustive descriptions of the herbs and their medicinal applications, the materia medica that follows focuses on medicine as an integrated view of well-being. Some of the language used in part 2 to describe medicinal uses of various plants is terminology common to Western herbalism. It is a kind of shorthand that conveys information but not spirit, and so falls short of shamanic truth. In keeping with a shamanic perspective, each herb listed herein is categorized in terms of elemental, directional, and/or planetary orientation, and the medicine of the plant is described through the herb's positive view of wellness.

Preparation notes give some idea of practical application, and the cautionary remarks at the end of some entries are reminders of wise relationship. Dosage ranges given here are moderate but not overly cautious; it is always best to start small with an unfamiliar herb and to consider individual factors, such as your tendency toward allergic reaction, general level of vitality, underlying conditions, and your weight and age. Some herbs are forgiving of overuse or misuse while others are not—as with foods and drugs, there is a wide spectrum of possible individual response to various herbs.

The herbs included in the materia medica were chosen because they are, for the most part, common plants—inexpensive to buy or easily found in North American habitats and, with some exceptions, are plants with which I am familiar. A few exotics, such as myrrh, copal, pau d'arco, and kava-kava, were included because they are widely used for medicinal and shamanic applications, yet not discussed in many classical texts.

Names for herbs can be confusing; Latin names are more standardized and specific than common names but can also vary from source to source. Some variation is due to official changes in nomenclature made over time, however, usually plants sharing a common name but different Latin names are different plants: American ginseng is not the same as Siberian ginseng, for example, even though both are commonly called *ginseng*. Closely related plants share a first name in Latin but have different last names, such as *Artemisia absinthium* (worm-wood) and *Artemisia vulgaris* (mugwort). Names can help you trace similarities and differences in plants as you become acquainted.

I leave it to you, the individual practitioner, to vitalize and expand on this information through your interaction with living plants. I hope that the heart and spirit of shamanic herbalism, represented in part 1, brings perspective and depth to the mind and body of herbalism, offered in part 2.

Aconite (*Aconitum napellus*) aka Monkshood, Wolfbane
Correspondences: West/Saturn/Water
Habitat: Aconite is a European perennial. Some species grow
wild in mountainous regions of the United States.
Parts used: The entire plant is used.
Plant characteristics and properties: Aconite offers freedom
from suffering through its treatment of feverish pain and
its use as a heart anodyne. The nature of aconite's freedom is that of unconventional or nonordinary reality,
which is why aconite is so often an ingredient in witches'
"flying ointments."
Preparation notes: Use in tincture form, 3–10 drops up to 4
times a day. Aconite is not to be used over an extended
period of time and should not be used by inexperienced
practitioners. *Aconite is toxic and can be lethal.*

Agrimony (*Agrimonia eupatoria*)
Correspondences: Southeast/Jupiter/Air
Habitat: Agrimony is a European native of shores and
ditches. It grows in thickets and woods of the northeast
and central United States.
Parts used: Aerial parts are used.
Plant characteristics and properties: Agrimony's medicine is
movement toward deeper integrity of consciousness. This
is demonstrated in its use as a liver herb—the liver being
associated with clarifying vision—and its quality of
drawing together (agrimony is used as an astringent for
childhood diarrhea). This herb eases muscles, heals
wounds, helps digestion, and is sometimes given for
appendicitis.
Preparation notes: Agrimony is usually taken in tincture
form, 20–30 drops 3 times a day, or as infusion, 3 to 4
times a day in small amounts.

Alfalfa *(Medicago sativa)*
Correspondences: North / Venus
Habitat: Widely cultivated, alfalfa grows in low valleys and field borders throughout much of the Unites States.
Parts used: The leaves are used.
Plant characteristics and properties: Alfalfa, with its extraordinary deep roots, offers the medicine of nourishment that comes from active, grounded seeking into universal resource. Alfalfa is rich in nutrients and enzymes. As a mild diuretic and appetite increaser, alfalfa encourages the flow of giving and receiving, and is a cooling bladder and kidney tonic.
Preparation notes: Alfalfa is taken raw, tinctured, or infused in small-cup doses. It is pleasant tasting and combines well with other herbs. Be careful of spoilage during the tincturing process.

Aloe *(Aloe vera)*
Correspondences: Northwest / Moon
Habitat: Aloe is a tropical growing perennial plant.
Parts used: The leaf gel is used.
Plant characteristics and properties: Aloe promotes integrity of surfaces and is an excellent burn remedy. It is also hung in doorways or planted on graves to aid in the maintenance of integrity during transitions. A bitter laxative, aloe urges cathartic clearing as an aspect of integrity. Aloe, though a tropical plant, is a cooling herb; it is itself regardless of context.
Preparation notes: Use aloe fresh or as a dehydrated juice. Combine 4 parts aloe powder with 1 part ginger root, in capsules, 2 caps 3 times a day, or apply raw gel externally. Avoid using aloe internally in situations of gastrointestinal inflammation, pregnancy, or lactation.

Angelica *(Angelica archangelica* or *A. sylvestris, A. atropurpurea, A. officinalis)*

Correspondences: Southeast / Venus / Sun

Habitat: Angelica favors damp meadows, riverbanks, and coastal areas in eastern North America and the midwest United States.

Parts used: The roots, leaves, and seeds are used.

Plant characteristics and properties: Angelica, through a nature that attracts goodness and encourages wisdom, gives little room for ill. It is used to prevent contagion, expel adherent placentas, clear lungs in feverish conditions, and discourage scabies and itching. Angelica relieves heartburn and hayfever, stimulates appetite, and, as a warming herb, promotes menses and perspiration. It is a positive, strong, and sweet presence.

Preparation notes: Use small doses of tincture (15–30 drops) or modest amounts (¹/₂–1 cup) of infusion. Angelica requires only a brief steeping. Avoid angelica in situations of pregnancy, high blood pressure, and diabetes.

Anise *(Pimpinella anisum)*

Correspondences: Southeast / Jupiter / Air

Habitat: An annual, anise is found wild but is mainly a cultivated plant.

Parts used: The seeds are used.

Plant characteristics and properties: Anise brings calmness to clear the path. It is an aromatic decongestant used for bronchitis and whooping cough; it expels gas, soothes the stomach, increases lactation, and helps movement in the dream and astral realms. Star anise, particularly, is useful in psychic work. Anise oil is employed for getting rid of lice and scabies. Anise is also used as a facial steam.

Preparation notes: Crush seeds and infuse, using 1–2 cups a day in mouthful doses. Alcohol extracts additional properties.

Balm *(Melissa officinalis)* aka Lemon Balm
Correspondences: Southwest/Moon
Habitat: A Mediterranean herb, balm has naturalized in North America. It can be found growing in fields and along roadsides.
Parts used: The leaves are used.
Plant characteristics and properties: Lemon balm's nature is gentle, cool, and assuring. Its medicine relieves cramps, colic, and mild fevers. Balm reduces stress and calms headaches; it is used in baths and sleep pillows for jumpy nerves and insomnia. As a tea herb, balm strengthens the solar plexus and revives the spirit. Like most herbs that attract honeybees, balm seems to attract love.
Preparation notes: Use fresh if possible, in tincture or infusion. Lemon balm is pleasant tasting and can be taken freely.

Balm of Gilead *(Populus candicans* or *P. gileadensis, P. balmsamifera)*
Correspondences: West/Venus/Water
Habitat: This tree is widely found in the eastern United States, Canada, and Alaska.
Parts used: The unopened buds are used.
Plant characteristics and properties: This tree medicine is concerned with healing externalized pain. It treats dry scaly skin eruptions, long-standing coughs, joint and muscle pain, and external inflammations. It is also given for laryngitis. These conditions give opportunity for addressing sources of unhappiness, with balm of Gilead as an ally.
Preparation notes: Water does not fully extract balm of Gilead, so tincture is used, 15–30 drops 3 to 4 times a day. For topical application, dilute the tincture with equal parts rubbing alcohol. Balm of Gilead is inappropriate to use in conjunction with anticoagulant therapy, or with

women who have an IUD. Do not use if there is kidney
disease, or sensitivity to aspirin.

Barberry *(Berberis vulgaris)*
Correspondences: West / Water
Habitat: Barberry is a shrub found in both the northeastern
and western United States. It grows in rich, gravely soil.
Parts used: The root, bark, and berries are used.
Plant characteristics and properties: Barberry operates with
a positive attitude. It is a liver tonic, promoting bile
secretion. Barberry urges forgiveness: it treats gallstones,
lowers blood pressure, reduces swollen spleen, relieves
hangovers and toxic effects from exposure to solvents.
Barberry is an antiseptic gargle, nurtures the gums, and is
used in the treatment of protozoan infections. Its berries
are refrigerant.
Preparation notes: Use barberry in a decoction, ½–1 cup a
day in 1-tablespoon doses, or take 10–60 drops of tincture
3 times a day. Conditions of liver disease, acute inflammations, or pregnancy contraindicate the use of barberry.

Basil *(Ocimum basilicum)*
Correspondences: Southeast / Mars
Habitat: Basil is indigenous to tropical and subtropical areas.
It is widely cultivated in North America.
Parts used: The aerial parts are used.
Plant characteristics and properties: Basil's medicine is
courage in the face of initiatory change and growth. It is a
funeral herb used for aiding the soul's journey and is
considered a holy plant in India. Basil helps bring on
menses and calms the stomach and head. Associated with
dragon energy, basil attracts prosperity and fertility, also
promoting lactation and perspiration. It is an herb of fluid
movement on many levels.

Preparation notes: Basil is best used fresh, as an infusion, 1–2 cups a day in mouthful doses.

Bayberry *(Myrica cerifera)*
Correspondences: Southwest
Habitat: Bayberry is an aromatic shrub growing over most of the United States.
Parts used: The bark and root are used.
Plant characteristics and properties: Bayberry is an herb of proportional or balanced wisdom within life's currents and flows. It is a circulatory tonic and is used to curtail menses, hemorrhage, prolapse, diarrhea, dysentery, colds, and varicosities. Bayberry's leaves and berries are macerated to make a liniment for sore joints and its bark is used as a douche for the uterus. Bayberry is considered a money totem.
Preparation notes: Use decoctions for astringency; use alcohol extractions for warming. Use either form in small doses (1 tablespoon) 3 times a day.

Belladonna *(Atropa belladonna)* aka Deadly Nightshade
Correspondences: West / Saturn
Habitat: Belladonna is a plant of waste places, pastures, and mountain forests.
Parts used: The leaves, tops, and berries are used.
Plant characteristics and properties: Belladonna's vision of life extends beyond constriction. It is an herb used for astral projection. Medicinally, belladonna is antispasmodic, diaphoretic, and diuretic; it is a homeopathic remedy for constrictive pains and ills of the nervous system.
Preparation notes: Use gloves when you gather this plant; its attributes can be absorbed through contact and cause toxic reactions. ***Belladonna is highly poisonous.*** It is not

to be used by inexperienced practitioners, except in homeopathic form.

Bethroot *(Trillium erectum* or *T. pendulum)*
Correspondences: Southeast
Habitat: Bethroot thrives in rich, shady forests of the middle United States and along the eastern seaboard into northeast Canada.
Parts used: The leaves and root are used.
Plant characteristics and properties: Bethroot speaks of the power of embodied, manifested life force. It contains precursors of female sex hormones and is used to start or strengthen labor contractions. An astringent, bethroot reduces all kinds of hemorrhage—postpartum, lung, menstrual flooding, and so on. It is also useful in treating ulcers and bronchial coughs.
Preparation notes: Use a decoction (1–2 cups daily in teaspoon doses), or tincture (15–25 drops) 3 times a day. Bethroot is inappropriate to use during pregnancy or in cases of acute inflammation.

Betony *(Stachyys officinalis* or *Betonica officinalis)* aka Wood Betony
Correspondences: North / Jupiter / Fire
Habitat: Betony can be found in moist areas of the Rocky Mountains.
Parts used: The flowering herb is used.
Plant characteristics and properties: Wood betony affirms mental and emotional equanimity. It strengthens the nervous system, eases headaches, reduces excessive sweating, and calms asthma or bronchitis. It is a purification herb used to banish nightmares or despair. Betony also relieves sprains and varicosities, reestablishing an experience of balance and well-being.

Preparation notes: Moderate daily amounts of infusion can be taken in mouthful doses. Betony can also be used in tincture form, 30 drops twice daily.

Blackberry *(Rubus villosus)*
Correspondences: East / Venus / Water
Habitat: Blackberry grows easily in dry, sandy areas and is widely cultivated.
Parts used: The leaves, fruit, and root bark are used.
Plant characteristics and properties: Blackberry takes a positive stance, causing the cessation and cooling of inconsiderate, irritated motion. Its medicine halts diarrhea, eases dysentery, and reduces hemorrhage. Blackberry treats leukorrhea and bleeding gums, and is used as a facial steam. As a nutrient tonic, blackberry is a protective ally.
Preparation notes: The leaf infusion is taken in daily ½–1 cup doses. Cold root-bark decoctions are taken 1–2 cups daily; root bark tincture is taken 15–40 drops as needed.

Black Cohosh *(Cimicifuga racemosa)*
Correspondences: East
Habitat: Hillsides and forests in the eastern United States are home to black cohosh.
Parts used: The root is used.
Plant characteristics and properties: Black cohosh is wise in matters of energetic pacing and cyclic balance. It is a uterine tonic—an estrogen herb—that clears pelvic congestion, brings on delayed menses, and normalizes circulation and blood pressure by depressing heart rate as it increases pulse strength. It addresses PMS and endometriosis and is a friend in times of constrictive stress—sedating nerves; calming asthma and bronchitis; easing dull, tense pains; and bringing relief during

headachy colds. Black cohosh is used for measles, whooping cough, and rheumatism, and is a traditional remedy for rattlesnake bites and other poisons.

Preparation notes: Use fresh or fresh dried roots; tinctures are preferred to decoctions. Use in small doses: 10–30 drops tincture or 1 tablespoon of cold decoction. Black cohosh should be avoided during pregnancy and lactation.

Black Haw *(Viburnum prunifolium)*
Correspondences: West
Habitat: Black haw grows in moist woodlands of the northeast, mid-Atlantic, and midwest United States.
Parts used: The root bark is used.
Plant characteristics and properties: Black haw's message is to relax and attune to a natural intelligence of timing and rhythm. This herb dispels false labor contractions and threatened miscarriages. It lowers blood pressure, eases cramping and pelvic pain, and lessens asthmatic spasms. Black haw is closely related to crampbark, and the two share similar natures.
Preparation notes: Use black haw in tincture form, 30–90 drops as needed, or in decoction, in 1-tablespoon doses as needed.

Blessed Thistle *(Carduus benedictus* or *Cerbenia benedicta)*
Correspondences: Northwest/Mars
Habitat: Native to Europe and Asia, blessed thistle is occasionally found wild in the United States.
Parts used: The aerial parts are used.
Plant characteristics and properties: Blessed thistle invokes and protects what strengthens life. It is used to induce vomiting of toxic substances and is antibacterial. It stimulates the appetites, and is a bitter, cooling tonic for liver and stomach. Blessed thistle encourages lactation and has

a positive effect on circulation. An herb associated in ancient times with Pan, protector and celebrator of life, blessed thistle continues to be an ally for bringing dreams into positive manifestation.

Preparation notes: Use in small doses, except as an emetic. The tincture dose is 5–20 drops as needed; blessed thistle can also be taken as an infusion, $^1/_2$ cup 3 times a day. Blessed thistle should not be used during pregnancy.

Blue Cohosh *(Caulophyllum thalictroides)*
Correspondences: Southwest
Habitat: Blue cohosh is found in wet areas of the eastern United States.
Parts used: The root is used.
Plant characteristics and properties: Blue cohosh's impulse is toward affirmative decision and action. Oxytocic in effect, blue cohosh stimulates labor contractions and menses and strongly inhibits postpartum bleeding. It treats chronic uterine or urinary inflammation and acts upon nervous disorders and rheumatism. A decisive herb, its direct properties are sometimes best utilized in combination with buffering herbs.
Preparation notes: Blue cohosh is used in tincture form, 5–20 drops as needed. Blue cohosh tends to irritate membranes, and so should be used in combination with other herbs. Be aware that blue cohosh will raise fetal heart rate and drop maternal blood pressure rate.

Boneset *(Eupatorium perfoliatum)*
Correspondences: Southwest/Saturn/Water
Habitat: Boneset is indigenous to the swampy areas of eastern North America.
Parts used: The aerial parts are used.
Plant characteristics and properties: Boneset deals with core

realities and the consequences of choice referent to those realities. It is used to treat bone weakness and muscular rheumatism of the bilious type. Boneset is also taken to alleviate night sweats, flu, colds, aches, congestion, and constipation. It is a bitter-tasting herb, associated with the liver, a good ally when seeking to look clearly beneath the distraction of symptoms.

Preparation notes: Large amounts of boneset are emetic. Take the infusion as hot as possible for flu, every half hour; drink warm infusion for fevers and cool infusion as a tonic. The tincture dose (10–40 drops) can be put into hot or cool water, as appropriate.

Borage *(Borago officinalis)*
Correspondences: Northwest/Jupiter/Air
Habitat: Borage is an annual from the Mediterranean countries. It is widely cultivated in North American gardens.
Parts used: The leaves and flowers are used.
Plant characteristics and properties: Borage is a gladdening herb, offering vitality, courage, and cheer during challenge. It strengthens the heart, revives adrenal glands, and is calmative and anti-inflammatory. Borage is steeped in wine to dispel melancholy; it is used as a bath herb for sore muscles and as a poultice for swellings. It is helpful during fever and lung ailments and will increase lactation. Borage used as a tea or amulet, or smoked, may enhance psychic ability.
Preparation notes: An infusion form is preferred, ¹/₂ cup 3 times a day.

Burdock *(Arctium lappa)*
Correspondences: Northwest/Venus
Habitat: Burdock thrives in waste places and roadsides of the northern United States and Europe.

Parts used: All plant parts are used.

Plant characteristics and properties: Deeply grounded, burdock is unfazed by adversity; it robustly hangs in when things get tough, and is unabashedly itself. Burdock neutralizes and eliminates substances that undermine health, working slowly and from the inside outward. It is particularly helpful in treatment of eczema and chronic skin eruptions, and clears heat and uric acid for relief of arthritis. Burdock is a nutritive blood tonic (root), kidney tonic (seeds), and a liver and skin tonic (fresh leaves) that also benefits the ovaries. Fresh leaves of burdock can be applied to poison oak or ivy.

Preparation notes: Long term use of burdock is best. Fresh root makes the best tincture (30–60 drops daily). The decoction dose is 1 cup daily.

Cactus *(Cactus grandiflorus* or *Selenicereus grandiforus* or *Cereus greggii)* aka Nightblooming Cereus

Correspondences: West

Habitat: Nightblooming cereus is a tropical plant of Mexico, the West Indies, and Naples. It is cutivated in Florida, and grows from southern Arizona to western Texas and northern Mexico.

Parts used: The flower is used.

Plant characteristics and properties: Nightblooming cereus expresses love's manifested nurturance and protection. This cactus is a superb cardiac tonic influencing the sympathetic nervous system. It is applied to functional abnormalities of the heart and treats palpitations, spasms, heart pain, anxiety, and fear of death. Nightblooming cereus is specific for nervous and tobacco-related heart problems. In small amounts it decreases pulse rate; it is sedative and diuretic. Other uses of this herb include treatment of pulmonary hemorrhage, interstitial pneumonia, and prostate or bladder irritations.

Preparation notes: Use this herb only in small doses. Tincture is made from fresh flowers and taken in 1–10 drop amounts.

Calendula *(Calendula officinalis)* aka Pot Marigold
Correspondences: Southeast
Habitat: Calendula is an annual; the garden is its usual habitat.
Parts used: The flowers are used.
Plant characteristics and properties: Calendula's primary perspective is of peace between inner and outer worlds. It is a comforting, cheering herb that heals ulcers, wounds, warts, rashes, bruises, colitis, varicosities, and skin conditions. Calendula soothes acid stomach and relieves cramps and diarrhea, and is an aid in stopping heavy bleeding. As a bath herb it will encourage perspiration, thereby lowering fevers. Its golden flowers are lightening to the spirit.
Preparation notes: Tincture in 5–20 drop doses is considered best for gastric problems. Fresh juice or infusion is preferred for most other situations. Steep the flowers for 5 to 10 minutes to make an infusion; when taken internally, use in frequent mouthful doses.

Cannabis *(Cannabis sativa)* aka Marijuana
Correspondences: West
Habitat: Cannabis is an annual indigenous to warm climate zones. It is widely cultivated.
Parts used: Flowering tops are used.
Plant characteristics and properties: Cannabis, an herb of sensual expansion, offers respite from mundane cares and expectations. It is euphorigenic, easing withdrawal from opiates and alcohol, and giving relief from chemotherapy nausea and migraine pain. Cannabis stimulates appetite;

it also promotes uterine contractions. It is antispasmodic,
antiepileptic, and antiasthmatic.

Preparation notes: This herb is usually smoked or added to
baked foods. It is easily overused by people reliant on
energy modifiers.

Catnip *(Nepeta cataria)*

Correspondences: Southwest/Venus

Habitat: Catnip grows wild in forests and waste places
throughout North America, and is often cultivated as a
garden herb.

Parts used: The aerial parts are used.

Plant characteristics and properties: Catnip acts in terms of
friendship between spirit and body. A gentle nervine,
catnip perks up the appetite and is itself nutritive. It
relaxes the digestive tract, easing colic, cramps, and
convulsions; is given for hysteria and headaches; and is
an excellent remedy for children's ills. Catnip's nature is
mellow and happy.

Preparation notes: Fresh catnip leaves are preferred for
infusion or tincture. The tincture dose is 30–40 drops 3
times a day. The infusion is taken cold as a tonic or hot as
a fever remedy, 1–2 cups daily.

Chamomile *(Anthemis nobilis* [Roman] or *Matricaria
chamomilla* [German]*)*

Correspondences: Southeast/Sun

Habitat: Chamomile favors dry fields and cultivated ground. It
is indigenous to southern Europe and has naturalized in
areas of North America having simiar growing conditions.

Parts used: The flowers are used.

Plant characteristics and properties: Chamomile, with its clear focus on life's blessings, is an herb applicable to many situations. Its action is mainly relieving and pacifying. Chamomile is used for cramps, stomach and intestinal distress, ulcers, insomnia, and irritable pain. It makes a good wash for eye inflammations or a douche for leukorrhea. Chamomile in homeopathic tablets is given for teething pain and startlement. The oil is used on swellings, bruises, and rashes. Other applications are as a tea for relief of menstrual congestion, as a poultice for earaches, or as a sitzbath for hemorrhoids.

Preparation notes: Steep infusion 5 to 10 minutes only. Large amounts taken at one time—2 cups infusion or the proportional amount of tincture— may cause vomiting.

Chaparral (*Larrea divericata*)

Correspondences: Northeast

Habitat: The arid deserts of the southwest are where to find chaparral.

Parts used: The leaves are used.

Plant characteristics and properties: Chaparral lends its aid when discernment fails, acting as a partisan helping to clear drug residues, metals, and radiation from the liver. Chaparral encourages bile production and aids fat metabolism; it is antibiotic, antioxidant, and antiseptic, and assists in the abatement of tumors. In addition to helping the liver, chaparral influences conditions involving the lymph. It is used to clear heat in the case of arthritis and is a remedy for parasitic infection.

Preparation notes: Chaparral is best used in tincture form. It is inappropriate for long-term use or use in large doses. The usual amount taken is 10–30 drops up to 3 times a day.

Chickweed (*Stellaria media*)

Correspondences: Northwest/Moon/Water

Habitat: Chickweed is found in abundance as a field and lawn weed throughout North America.

Parts used: The aerial parts are used.

Plant characteristics and properties: Chickweed's gentle medicine is renewal within connectedness. It relieves irritations such as eczema and itching, healing digestive upsets and bowel ulcers. Chickweed is an excellent remedy for eye inflammations, and it soothingly cools sores, bruises, and hemorrhoids. A salad herb, chickweed is diuretic and laxative, relieving constipation. It is also taken to dissolve cysts.

Preparation notes: Use chickweed raw, or simmer the fresh herb for 30 minutes and use in small cup doses. Tincture should be made from the fresh herb; use ¹/₂-teaspoon doses as needed. Avoid chickweed during pregnancy, except in small amounts.

Chicory (*Cichorium intybus*)

Correspondences: Southeast/Sun

Habitat: Chicory graces the roadsides of the United States, Canada, and Europe.

Parts used: The roots, leaves, and flowers are used.

Plant characteristics and properties: Chicory's perspective is the awakening of insight. In esoteric reference it is associated with psychic vision, dissolution of obstacles, and invisibility. It urges transcendence, not avoidance. Supportive of the liver, spleen, and gall bladder, chicory is a remedy for jaundice. It is also used to benefit the glandular aspect of digestion, and is a remedy for eye inflammations.

Preparation notes: Chicory is taken as an infusion or decoction, 1–2 cups a day.

Cinquefoil *(Potentilla anserina* or *P. simplex, P. tormentilla, P. canadensis)*

Correspondences: Southwest/Jupiter

Habitat: Cinquefoil, found in meadows and marshes, is common to much of the United States and Europe.

Parts used: The aerial parts are used.

Plant characteristics and properties: Used with awareness, cinquefoil magnetizes appropriate energies. It is considered an ally for movement through astral realms, a household protector, and an aid to prophetic dreaming. Medicinally, it is an astringent used for bacterial infections, sore throats and gums, skin disturbances, feverish flu, and diarrhea. It has been noted that frogs like to sit under cinquefoil plants.

Preparation notes: The infusion dose is 1 cup a day. Cinquefoil can also be taken in tincture form, 20–40 drops at a time. Use fresh plant parts for tincturing or infusion.

Coltsfoot *(Tussilago farfara)*

Correspondences: East/Venus/Water

Habitat: Coltsfoot prefers wet areas and embankments of loamy or limestone soils in eastern North America.

Parts used: The aerial parts are used.

Plant characteristics and properties: Coltsfoot has an accepting and tranquil nature, yet contains an astringency that keeps things together. As an antispasmodic, coltsfoot is useful for coughs, colds, and asthma; its astringent quality is healing to bites, boils, and abscesses.

Preparation notes: The tincture dosage is 30–60 drops as needed. Hot infusion can be taken $^1/_2$-cup doses 3 times a day; coltsfoot can also be taken in the form of fresh juice in the same $^1/_2$-cup doses. Dried coltsfoot leaves can be smoked.

Comfrey *(Symphytum officinale)*
Correspondences: West/Saturn
Habitat: Comfrey thrives in moist areas and is easily
   propagated.
Parts used: The root and leaves are used.
Plant characteristics and properties: Comfrey champions
   proliferant participation; adversity encourages its medicine
   of regeneration and reconnection. Comfrey heals wounds,
   sprains, and breakage. The root is a demulcent for peptic
   ulcers, dry coughs, and coughs with blood. Comfrey is
   vigorously nutritive. It is healing to kidneys, bladder,
   intestines, and pancreas, and is often used as a douche or
   sitzbath, or a poultice for bruises, cuts, and tears.
Preparation notes: Fresh tinctured comfrey is preferred, 20–
   30 drops 3 times a day. Comfrey can also be used raw or
   fresh infused/decocted. Leaf infusion of comfrey spoils
   easily. Avoid comfrey in situations of liver disease, deep
   wounds in their early stages, or dysplasia.

Cornsilk *(Zea mays)*
Correspondences: Southwest/Venus/Earth
Habitat: Corn is widely cultivated throughout much of North
   America and Central America.
Parts used: The stigmas from female flowers are used.
Plant characteristics and properties: Cornsilk is a refinement
   of earthiness. A diuretic and antiseptic, cornsilk neutral-
   izes excess alkalinity in urine, clears away urea, and
   comforts the kidneys and bladder. It is an herb with none
   of the harshness found in many diuretics.
Preparation notes: Use fresh silk while the plant is still green.
   Infusions steep 5 to 15 minutes; use 1 cup daily, 3 times a
   day. Tincture dosage is 5–20 drops as needed.

Crampbark *(Viburnum opulus)*
Correspondences: Southwest
Habitat: Crampbark prefers moist forests and thickets in
eastern North America.
Parts used: The bark is used.
Plant characteristics and properties: Crampbark offers an
affirmative warmth and ease in its release from constriction. It relaxes menstrual and postpartum cramps and
helps prevent miscarriage. Crampbark also reduces
menopausal bleeding. A nervine, this herb quiets heart
palpitations, helps with PMS, and diminishes spasms of
the stomach, gall bladder, lungs, jaw, rectum, and
muscles. It is part of the elder family and is related to
black haw.
Preparation notes: Use fresh or dried bark, preferably in
tincture form, 20–90 drops every few hours as needed.
For decoction, simmer 15 minutes; use in 1-tablespoon
doses as needed. Crampbark should not be used for more
than three consecutive days.

Damiana *(Turnera diffusa* or *T. aphrodisiaca)*
Correspondences: Southwest / Mars
Habitat: Damiana is at home in the dry areas of the southwest and Mexico.
Parts used: The leaves are used.
Plant characteristics and properties: Damiana's nature is allied
with the sacred fire within. It is a tonic for sexual debility
and is antidepressant. Damiana enlivens the appetite,
strengthens the nerves, and has a testosterone-like action. It
is sometimes smoked to invoke dreams and visions.
Preparation notes: The infusion dose is 1 cup 3 times a day;
tincture dose is 30–60 drops 1 to 2 times a day. Damiana is
inappropriate in situations of pregnancy, inflammation,
or overt pathology.

Dandelion *(Taraxacum officinale)*
Correspondences: East / Sun / Jupiter
Habitat: Dandelion is a perennial found throughout North
    America; it is a prolific lawn weed.
Parts used: All plant parts are used.
Plant characteristics and properties: Dandelion offers
    abundant good wishes. Its orientation is to strong
    beginnings and vigorous flow. Medicinally, dandelion
    has wide application. It is highly nutritive, tones the
    body's organs and passages, and stimulates the pan-
    creas, spleen, and kidneys. The urinary system and liver
    benefit from dandelion. It lowers cholesterol, prevents
    anemia and jaundice, is a diuretic for heart conditions,
    and is used for treating toxemia, diabetes, hypo-glyce-
    mia, gallstones, rheumatism, and deep-seated skin
    problems. Dandelion sap is applied to warts. This
    versatile herb is also associated with spirit-calling,
    divination, and weather magic.
Preparation notes: Fresh tincture or decoction is preferred
    (shake before use). Raw young leaves are good in salads;
    older leaves are more medicinal. Administer decoctions
    cold. Long-term use is most effective; the dosage is 30–
    90 drops of tincture 2 times a day. Dandelion is inappro-
    priate when there is acute inflammation.

Datura *(Datura discolor* or *D. stramonium, D. innoxia)*
Correspondences: West / Saturn
Habitat: Considered a pest plant, datura grows in waste
    areas, pastures, and fields.
Parts used: The leaves are used.
Plant characteristics and properties: Datura's medicine
    disrupts the continuity of habitual patterning, though
    used unwisely it allows chaos to become a pattern in
    itself. Datura is hallucinogenic, narcotic, and sedative,

having the same alkaloids (atropine and scopolamine) as deadly nightshade.

Preparation notes: Datura is smoked or ingested. Mexican datura is stronger than American datura, but *both are poisonous, and not for casual use.*

Dittany of Crete *(Origanum dictamnus* or *Cunila origanoides)*
Correspondences: West / Venus / Water
Habitat: Naturalized from gardens, dittany grows in clearings and forest openings from the midwestern states to New York and Pennsylvania.
Parts used: The leaves are used.
Plant characteristics and properties: Dittany's nature is projective. It is an ally of astral travel and is used as a magical incense. Part of the mint family, dittany is not oft-used medicinally but does have the effect of increasing lactation.
Preparation notes: Dittany is most commonly used in incense form.

Devil's Club *(Oplopanax horridum)*
Correspondences: West
Habitat: Lakesides and mountainsides of the Pacific Northwest are home to devil's club.
Parts used: The root bark is used.
Plant characteristics and properties: Devil's club confronts ill with a perspective of cohesion. It is a strongly adaptogenic herb having a modifying effect on the limbic system. It treats such conditions as schizophrenia, kidney and liver illness, and type II insulin-resistant diabetes. This herb is considered a powerful ally by northwest Native healers.
Preparation notes: Tincture dose is 10–30 drops up to 4 times a day. Avoid devil's club during pregnancy.

Echinacea (*Echinacea augustifolia* or *E. purpurea*)
Correspondences: Northeast
Habitat: Echinacea is indigenous to the northeastern United States and the prairies of the midwest.
Parts used: The root is the primary part used, although leaves and flowers are also used.
Plant characteristics and properties: Echinacea asserts integrity amid negative influences, affirming the strength of natural, harmonious function. The immune system is stimulated by echinacea, which contains polysaccharides that affect white blood cells and the surface chemistry of cells. An antimicrobial, echinacea is used for viral, bacterial, and fungal infections and is disease preventive. It also treats bites, stings, poison ivy and oak, and blood poisoning.
Preparation notes: Decoct or tincture using fresh roots; polysaccharides are mostly water soluble, so fresh decoction can be added to tincture for added potency. Use for 7 to 10 days at a time in small, frequent amounts—20–60 drops tincture or 1-tablespoon decoction doses.

Elder (*Sambucus canadensis* or *S. nigra*)
Correspondences: Southwest/Venus
Habitat: Elder favors wetland areas. It is widely found in the northeastern and central parts of the United States.
Parts used: The berries, leaves, flowers, bark, and root are used.
Plant characteristics and properties: Elder's nature is discerning, discriminating, and protective. Used warm, elder reduces fevers; taken cold, it is diuretic. Elder treats colds,

hayfever, and other autumnal, watery conditions. In topical application it soothes sunburn and abrasions. The flowers make an excellent tea for children's fevers; leafbuds are purgative and diuretic; the root is diuretic. Dried or cooked berries in cold infusion treat diarrhea and hayfever. A hot infusion purges boils or splinters.

Preparation notes: Tincture the flowers fresh; dry other parts before use. Tincture dose is 15–30 drops 3 times a day. Dwarf elderberries and red or blue elder seeds are poisonous.

Elecampane *(Inula helenium)*

Correspondences: Northeast/Mercury

Habitat: Elecampane is a tall perennial of roadsides and fields. It can be found from Ontario and Nova Scotia southward.

Parts used: The root is used.

Plant characteristics and properties: Elecampane brings a healthy continuity between realms—an endurance of vital essence. It is associated with rites of initiation, psychic power, divination, and elves. Elecampane's primary medicinal use is for chronic lung problems, chest congestion, and bronchial infection; it is not as effective for dry coughs, but warms and strengthens the lungs. Other uses include application as a wash for scabies and itches or a facial steam for skin disturbances, and as a tonic for digestion. Elecampane is astringent and antiseptic.

Preparation notes: Use a cold decoction or tincture that is slightly heated before administering; tincture dose is 20–50 drops 3 times a day, or use 1–2 cups daily of decoction in 1 tablespoon doses.

Eyebright *(Euphrasia officinalis)*
Correspondences: East/Sun
Habitat: Eyebright is common to grassy areas in Europe and
   Asia and is naturalized in some areas of the United States,
   including New England, and in Newfoundland.
Parts used: Aerial parts are used.
Plant characteristics and properties: Clarity of thought and
   vision characterize eyebright, a joyful herb used to remedy photosensitivity, poor sight, and eye ailments of all
   kinds, acute or chronic. Eyebright has an astringent effect
   on hayfever, sinusitis, head colds, and lung problems,
   and is used in treatment of allergies. It stimulates the liver
   and aids thought and memory. Eyebright is a traditional
   cleansing fluid for scrying devices.
Preparation notes: Eyebright is best tinctured fresh and given
   in small, frequent doses (4 to 6 times a day). It can also be
   taken as an infusion 3 times a day.

False Unicorn *(Chamealirium luteum)*
Correspondences: Southwest
Habitat: Moist woodlands and meadows in the south, east,
   and midland states are where this plant can be found.
Parts used: The root is used.
Plant characteristics and properties: False unicorn reflects a
   readiness to embrace fertility and manifestation. It contains precursors of estrogen, which help normalize
   menses and reproductive function. False unicorn is a
   uterine and reproductive tonic and is sometimes used to
   help prevent miscarriage.
Preparation notes: Decoction or tincture is used 3 times a day
   in small doses—15–30 drops tincture or ¹/₂ cup decoction
   3 times a day. For threatened miscarriage, use liberally—
   15 drops tincture every hour.

Fennel *(Foeniculum vulgare)*
Correspondences: Southeast/Mercury
Habitat: Fennel is indigenous to the Mediterranean and Asia Minor, and is common to gardens elsewhere.
Parts used: The seeds are used.
Plant characteristics and properties: Fennel offers a purifying strength within adversity, invoking core virtues. Often taken to relieve cramps of the stomach, bowel, or uterus, fennel also clears mucus congestion and promotes lactation. It reduces appetite and is a good ally when fasting. Fennel is also taken as a brain tonic and is used as a facial steam.
Preparation notes: Infusion or tincture are taken as needed. Tincture dose is 10–30 drops.

Fenugreek *(Trigonella foenum-graecum)*
Correspondences: Northwest/Air
Habitat: Fenugreek is a Middle Eastern annual, widely cultivated.
Parts used: The seeds are used.
Plant characteristics and properties: Fenugreek has a congenial nature conducive to positive interaction and interface. Its mucilaginous seeds soothe the stomach and intestines and alleviate fevers and bronchitis. Fenugreek makes a good poultice for boils and infections; it gives strength to invalids with its nutrient qualities, and promotes fertility and lactation. Fenugreek is also known to attract prosperity.
Preparation notes: Use as a decoction, 1 cup daily, or in tincture form, 30–60 drops 3 times a day.

Feverfew *(Chrysanthemum parthenium* or *Pyrethrum parthenium)*

Correspondences: Southwest/Venus/Water

Habitat: Feverfew is found on roadsides and waste places mainly in the eastern half of North America.

Parts used: The leaves and flowers are used.

Plant characteristics and properties: Feverfew offers a centered response to stress. It inhibits prostaglandin biosynthesis, so is used for PMS or migraine headaches and in the treatment of fevers, colds, and flu. It eases asthma, bronchitis, and arthritis. Warm infusions of feverfew leaves relieve nervousness and alcoholic DTs. Used cold, feverfew is a digestive and intestinal tonic.

Preparation notes: Use as a tincture or an infusion—fresh leaves are needed for both. (Commercial feverfew preparations are often in the form of freeze-dried leaves packaged as tablets or capsules.) The infusion dose is 1–2 cups daily in mouthful amounts, or 10–30 drops tincture (tincture is preferred). Regular, long-term use is necessary for effective treatment of migraine pain, however, some users experience side effects, such as mouth ulcers, abdominal pain, and indigestion, from regular use. The flowers are purgative. Do not use feverfew during pregnancy, and discontinue use in the event of side effects.

Garlic *(Allium sativum)*

Correspondences: South/Mars

Habitat: Garlic is commonly cultivated as a culinary herb.

Parts used: The bulb is used.

Plant characteristics and properties: Garlic believes in living well through the wise use of will and desire. It has a crone's sexual energy. Garlic helps prevent and treat infections; it supports beneficial digestive bacteria, lowers blood cholesterol, normalizes blood pressure, and is good for the liver and gall bladder. Another primary use of garlic is as a vermifuge for threadworms, pinworms, and ringworms. Its antiseptic properties are employed for cleansing wounds and treating colds.

Preparation notes: Use juice, raw cloves, tincture (10–30 drops), or cold infusion 3 times a day as needed. Raw juice will burn skin or sensitive membranes—use with care.

Gentian *(Gentiana lutea or G. catesbaei or Swertia radiata)*
Correspondences: Northeast / Mars / Fire
Habitat: All gentians prefer wetland habitat.
Parts used: The root is used.
Plant characteristics and properties: Gentian urges assimilation and positive movement. Sluggishness and lack of appetite are dispelled. Gentian is a bitter digestive tonic; it is also antiseptic and an emmenagogue. The root of gentian is chewed to discourage smoking; it can also be added to baths or sachets to promote love. Gentian is also an herb employed for breaking curses.
Preparation notes: One-quarter cup of decoction or 5–15 drops of tincture are taken ten minutes before meals. Gentian is inappropriate in situations of acute gastrointestinal inflammation.

Ginger *(Zingiber officinalis* [Jamaican, considered best] or *Asarum canadensis* [wild, American]*)*
Correspondences: South / Mars
Habitat: Ginger is a tropical Asian plant whose American counterpart grows in rich soil near streams and lakes.
Parts used: The root is used.
Plant characteristics and properties: Ginger's hot, first-chakra energy is given to the activation and circulation of vitality. This herb has a grounded intensity that both catalyzes and comforts irritated systems. It alleviates nausea, morning sickness, and motion sickness, and

encourages menses that is delayed by cold. Ginger stimulates circulation and digestion, promotes sweating, and is
a warming footbath that helps fevers and phlegmatic
conditions.

Preparation notes: Use tea from powder, or a heated decoction ($^1/_2$ cup), or tincture (10–20 drops) as needed.

Ginseng *(Panax quinquefolius* [wild, American] or
Eleutherococcus senticosus [Siberian])

Correspondences: Southeast/Sun

Habitat: Ginseng requires damp, cool, rich-soiled woodlands.

Parts used: The root is used.

Plant characteristics and properties: Ginseng amplifies
perspective of capacity, and conveys this through its
medicine. Ginseng is a tonic for increasing performance;
it stimulates and rejuvenates. Digestive and adrenal
glands are catalyzed by ginseng. The cured, red Chinese
and Korean ginsengs tend to be hypertensive and hy-
poglycemic—"hotter" than Siberian or uncured, white
Asian and American ginsengs. The various types have
differing medicinal properties.

Preparation notes: Ginseng can be chewed raw, decocted,
or tinctured; use small amounts over a long term.
Ginseng is inappropriate during pregnancy and in
situations of steroid therapy, hypoglycemia, hyperthyroid, hyper-andrenocortical conditions, or other major
pathologies.

Goldenrod *(Solidago virgauria* or *S. odora)*

Correspondences: Northeast/Venus/Air

Habitat: Goldenrod, a common field perennial of the eastern
half of the United States, grows in dry sandy soil.

Parts used: Aerial parts are used.

Plant characteristics and properties: Goldenrod's outlook is confident yet flexible, urging positive acceptance of change. Tonic to the kidneys and a bladder astringent, goldenrod also treats acute or chronic upper respiratory congestion and laryngitis. It is a supportive herb in remedies for flu, and the crushed fresh leaves help relieve stings and wounds. Goldenrod is traditionally considered an herb of prosperity.

Preparation notes: Tincture or infuse goldenrod fresh. It can be taken 3 times a day. Exercise care with goldenrod if you have pollen allergies.

Goldenseal *(Hydrastis canadensis)*
Correspondences: Northeast / Sun / Fire
Habitat: Goldenseal thrives in rich soil and dappled shade.
Parts used: The root is used.
Plant characteristics and properties: Goldenseal is involved with an immediacy of engagement and vulnerability. It is a wisdom teacher. Goldenseal heals body surfaces. It is taken as an antibiotic for sinus infections and colds and is used as an antiseptic tonic for gastrointestinal mucous membranes. Goldenseal is an effective wash for sores, gum abscesses, shallow wounds, and eye infections. It is a tonic for most digestive disorders and strengthens the heart muscle. Though cooling, goldenseal stimulates the heart and respiration. Chickenpox, measles, and ring-worm are also treated with goldenseal. Careful discern-ment should be used with this ally, however—goldenseal disturbs balances of beneficial bacteria, thereby weaken-ing the immune system and allowing yeast overgrowths.

Preparation notes: Make the tincture from dried root; fresh root tends to cause ulcerative membrane conditions. Use goldenseal in small doses as powder or tincture—20–50 drops of tincture up to 4 times a day for 7 to 10 days. Goldenseal is inappropriate during pregnancy, or in situations of liver or kidney disease or acute infection.

Hawthorne *(Crataegus oxyacantha)*
Correspondences: South/Mars
Habitat: Hawthorne grows as a shrub or tree. It is indigenous
  to England and North Africa.
Parts used: The berries, leaves, and flowers are used.
Plant characteristics and properties: Hawthorne is character-
  ized by a sense of joyful renewal, a loving participation in
  life grounded in being true to oneself. A well-beloved
  heart tonic, hawthorne strengthens the heart's rhythm,
  treats arteriosclerosis and angina, and normalizes blood
  pressure. It is helpful in dealing with stress and insomnia,
  is diuretic, and has an astringent effect on sore throats.
  Hawthorne, associated with chastity, is an herb sacred to
  the Little People.
Preparation notes: Long-term use of hawthorne is necessary
  for results. Use as an infusion, 1 cup 3 times a day, or in
  tincture form, 10–30 drops 3 times a day. Avoid
  hawthorne if you are taking beta blockers or have bradycardia conditions.

Henbane *(Hyoscyamus niger)*
Correspondences: Northwest/Saturn/Water
Habitat: Henbane favors waste places, cemeteries, and dry,
  sandy soil around old house foundations.
Parts used: The aerial parts are used.
Plant characteristics and properties: Henbane destructures the
  notion of limited reality. It is similar to nightshade and
  datura but less extreme. It is an herb that brings you face to
  face with your fears and beliefs. Henbane is narcotic; it is
  used in witches' "flying ointments." It allays pain, insomnia, and nervousness. Henbane is antispasmodic and
  calmative but can also produce convulsions and death. It
  has been used medicinally as a remedy for lice.
Preparation notes: Henbane is smoked or used externally in
  decoction. *It is highly poisonous and can be fatal.*

Hops *(Humulus lupulus)*
Correspondences: North / Mars / Air
Habitat: Hop vines are mainly found cultivated.
Parts used: The female flowers and fruit are used.
Plant characteristics and properties: Hops is an ally of self-referent restoration, of introverted calm. It is a nervine and sedative for insomnia, restlessness, agitation, and nervous stomach. Hops increases appetite and lactation; it is used to alleviate cramping and gas and as a wash for boils and rashes, utilizing its antiseptic and astringent properties.
Preparation notes: Hops is taken fresh, tinctured or infused. Tincture dose is 30–60 drops as needed. Hops should not be used over extended periods of time, and is inappropriate with depression.

Horehound *(Marrubium vulgare)*
Correspondences: Southeast / Mercury
Habitat: Horehound grows in pastures and coastal zones of North America and Mexico.
Parts used: The leaves are used.
Plant characteristics and properties: Horehound brings clarity to the aura. It is an herb of mental and emotional openness and creativity. Familiar as a remedy for lung congestion, horehound is particularly healing for dry coughs, smoker's coughs, and sore throats. It is mildly laxative and a good herb to use when preparing to fast. Horehound calms heart action, has been used for treating typhoid fever, and is a beneficial skin wash.
Preparation notes: Horehound can be smoked, or used in infusion (1 cup daily). Tincture dose is 30–60 drops 3 times a day. Horehound can also be taken in syrup.

Horsetail *(Equisetum arvense)*
Correspondences: Southwest / Saturn / Earth
Habitat: Horsetail thrives along streambanks and wet
    shady areas. It ranges over almost the entire Northern
    hemisphere.
Parts used: The aerial parts are used.
Plant characteristics and properties: Horsetail embodies
    positive ancestral patterns of structure and growth. It is
    an herb rich in silica and calcium, and is astringent and
    diuretic. Horsetail is taken for bladder and kidney ills,
    also treating prostate inflammation or benign enlarge-
    ment. It alleviates bedwetting, helps coagulate blood, and
    calms the liver. Horsetail can also be used as a wash for
    wounds, eczema, sores, and boils. In some cultures it is an
    herb associated with snake charming.
Preparation notes: Use horsetail fresh (early stems only), as
    an infusion, in mouthful doses; or in tincture form, 30–60
    drops, up to 4 times a day. Avoid prolonged use, or in
    cases of continued inflammation.

Hyssop *(Hyssopus officinale)*
Correspondences: Southeast / Jupiter / Fire
Habitat: Hyssop is native to southern Europe and is grown
    as a garden herb in the United States
Parts used: The aerial parts are used.
Plant characteristics and properties: The power of innocence
    is expressed by hyssop. An herb long associated with
    purification and protection, it is medicinally applied to
    children's ills, coughs, colds, and lingering fevers.
    Hyssop's energy is warm and mild. It calms anxiety and
    is used topically for bruises, cuts, rashes, and nerve pain.
Preparation notes: The infusion dose is ¹/₂ cup 3 times a day.
    In tincture form, take 30–60 drops 3 times a day. Hyssop
    is inappropriate for extended use.

Irish Moss (*Chondrus crispus*)
Correspondences: West/Moon/Water
Habitat: Irish moss is a seaweed found on underwater rocks off the coasts of France and Ireland.
Parts used: All parts are used.
Plant characteristics and properties: Irish moss gracefully attunes to cycles and flows. A nurturant herb, the demulcent quality of Irish moss soothes respiratory ills, such as tuberculosis, coughs, and bronchitis. This nutritive seaweed cools ulcers, soothes the skin, and comforts the kidneys. Considered a lucky herb, Irish moss is carried for protection during travels.
Preparation notes: Decoction dose is 1–2 cups daily.

Juniper (*Juniperis communis*)
Correspondences: Southwest/Sun/Fire
Habitat: Juniper is widely found growing in dry, rocky soil in North America, Europe, and Asia.
Parts used: The berries are used.
Plant characteristics and properties: Juniper embodies creative acceptance and perseverance, embodying a kind of soul alchemy, a purifying beauty. Juniper is used as a remedy for cystitis and gravel, and for rheumatism, arthritis, and joint pain. It is antiseptic and diuretic, considered an herb of protection and clearing. Juniper relieves colic and supports digestion.
Preparation notes: The infusion dose is 1–2 cups daily; use 10–20 drops of juniper tincture 3 times a day. Juniper is inappropriate in situations of pregnancy, kidney disease, acute cystitis, or gastric inflammation. Juniper should not be used on a long-term basis.

Kava-Kava *(Piper methysticum)*
Correspondences: East / Saturn / Water
Habitat: Kava-kava is native to the South Sea Islands.
Parts used: The root is used.
Plant characteristics and properties: Kava-kava shifts outlook.
   It raises the pain threshold and is a sedative used for
   dreaming and visions. Specific for treating periodic peptic
   ulcer pain and congested urinary inflammation, kava-kava
   is also used for gastritis and cystitis, and may be helpful for
   arthritis. In small doses it has a stimulant effect. Generally
   antiseptic and used in the treatment of sexually transmitted
   diseases, kava-kava is also an aphrodisiac.
Preparation notes: Kava-kava can be taken in decoction or
   tincture. The tincture dose is 20–40 drops 4 times a day
   for cystitis, or 15–25 drops 4 times a day for gastritis. Use
   kava-kava carefully; large amounts can damage kidneys,
   liver, and respiration.

Lavender *(Lavendula officinalis)*
Correspondences: East / Mercury
Habitat: Lavender is a Mediterranean shrub now widely
   cultivated for its flowers.
Parts used: The flowers are used.
Plant characteristics and properties: Lavender clears the
   path on which blessings flow. It is an herb of love, joy,
   peace, and long life. Lavender eases stress headaches,
   nervous exhaustion, and insomnia. An antiseptic, it is
   strengthening to the nerves, metabolism, and immune
   system. Lavender is a clearing wash for skin disturbances; its gentle fragrance underlies a surprising
   strength and effectiveness. Lavender, ally of birth, dem-
   onstrates clarity and power within nurturance and alignment to love.
Preparation notes: Sometimes the leaves are infused, but
   most often the flowers are used externally or internally,

often in oil form for external application. Infusion dose is
$^{1}/_{2}$–1 cup a day.

Licorice *(Glycyrrhiza glabra)*
Correspondences: Northwest / Venus / Water
Habitat: Indigenous to Europe and Asia, licorice is widely
  cultivated elsewhere.
Parts used: The root is used.
Plant characteristics and properties: Licorice encourages the
  renewability of expressive freedom. An herb long associated with love and with both lust and fidelity, licorice has
  an estrogenic and steroidal action. It is used to remedy
  infertility and irregular menses, and as an ally during
  menopause. Licorice is demulcent and laxative. It relieves
  peptic ulcers, congestion, coughs, bronchitis, and laryngitis. The liver and adrenal glands benefit from use of
  licorice, and it is also helpful in treating lupus.
Preparation notes: Decoction is taken in 1-tablespoon doses;
  the tincture is taken in doses of 30–60 drops 3 times a day.
  Licorice is inappropriate in situations of pregnancy,
  edema, or steroid use.

Linden *(Tilia europa* or *T. americana)*
Correspondences: East / Jupiter / Air
Habitat: Linden or European lime *(Tilia europa)* or basswood
  (T. americana) is a tree of forest and mountains. American
  basswood is found in the Canadian Maritimes, New
  England, and the midwest.
Parts used: The flowers are used.
Plant characteristics and properties: Linden sweetly shelters
  as it urges calmness and expansion. It is specific for
  feverish colds and flu, and also protects against arterio-
  sclerosis and high blood pressure. Linden may help with
  some migraines; it relaxes nervous tension, offering

respite in which choices and changes can be considered.

Preparation notes: Infusion dose is 1 cup a day; linden can also be taken in tincture form, 30–45 drops 2 times a day. It is inappropriate for long term use, which can damage the heart.

Lobelia (*Lobelia inflata*)

Correspondences: West / Saturn / Water

Habitat: Lobelia is native to North American pastures and fields, growing in the northeastern and north central United States.

Parts used: Aerial parts are used.

Plant characteristics and properties: Lobelia deals in conflict resolution; its perspective is one of situational wisdom. It is a paradoxical herb—extremely dose sensitive—it is antispasmodic in small amounts and emetic in large doses. Lobelia is both a respiratory stimulant and relaxant, used for asthma, bronchitis, whooping cough, and pneumonia. Earaches and tetanus are treated with lobelia. It has a tendency to equalize circulation (and is associated with halting storms). Used as a bath herb, lobelia may help ease muscle spasms.

Preparation notes: Sometimes lobelia is smoked. It is also used in tincture form, 5–15 drops, for relaxing the nervous system. Use lobelia briefly and carefully. It is inappropriate in situations of shock, paralysis, gangrene, or bradycardia.

Mandrake (*Podophyllum peltatum* [American] or *Mandragora officinarum* [European])

Correspondences: Northeast / Mercury / Fire

Habitat: Mandrake is a perennial of the open woodlands. It can be found in Ontario, New England, and parts of the midwest.

Plant characteristics and properties: Mandrake serves well-being through divestment and radical change. American mandrake is cathartic; it is used for chronic digestive problems and to stimulate the glands, liver, and gall bladder. European mandrake is emetic and purgative, and an anesthetic for pain and melancholy. Mandrake is ceremonially used to amplify power and provide protective presence.

Preparation notes: Decoction dose is 1 teaspoon; tincture dose is 1–15 drops 2 times a day. Avoid mandrake during pregnancy. Mandrake should only be used by experienced practitioners. *Both American and European mandrake are considered poisonous.*

Marshmallow *(Althaea officinalis)*
Correspondences: West
Habitat: Marshmallow is found in wetlands and swamps from Connecticut to Virginia and locally inland.
Parts used: The root, leaves, and flowers are used.
Plant characteristics and properties: Marshmallow believes in minimizing friction. It transforms provocation with its cool, mild, sweet nature, soothing the skin and digestive tract with its demulcent root and offering comfort to respiratory and urinary passages with its leaves. Marshmallow relieves congestion and inflammation; it is a gentle wash for abscesses and varicosities. Marshmallow lubricates, and also promotes lactation.
Preparation notes: Decoction or infusion of marshmallow can be used in 1-cup dosages, 3 times a day. Tincture dosage is 30–60 drops 3 times a day.

Milk Thistle *(Silybum marianum or Carduus marianum)*
Correspondences: Northeast/Mars/Fire
Habitat: Milk thistle grows in rocky, dry soils, mainly in

Europe but also in some areas of the United States.

Parts used: The seeds are used.

Plant characteristics and properties: Milk thistle gives persevering attention. It urges taking responsibility for well-being—making wise choices, but with a compassion that allows renewal. Milk thistle heals chronic and acute liver illness: cirrhosis, hepatitis, mushroom poisoning, solvent and chemical poisoning, and the effects of alcoholism. It increases bile flow and benefits the gall bladder and spleen. The leaves are a bitter tonic for the stomach. Milk thistle is also a remedy useful in treating varicose veins.

Preparation notes: Tincture is the preferred form for use, in doses of 15–25 drops 4 times a day.

Motherwort *(Leonurus cardiaca)*

Correspondences: West

Habitat: Motherwort can be found along fences, paths, and in waste places in the northern United States and Europe.

Parts used: The flowering tops are used.

Plant characteristics and properties: Motherwort's nature is supportive of love and acceptance. This herb promotes normal heart action, reducing tachycardia and hypertension when used in cold infusion. Used warm, motherwort encourages menses, relieves chronic pain and cramping, and also increases lactation. It acts as a mellowing nervine to ease anxiety, tension, and melancholy.

Preparation notes: Use a cold infusion or tincture for the heart. Tincture dose is 15–40 drops 2 to 3 times a day. Be careful of skin reaction when harvesting motherwort. Avoid motherwort during pregnancy, in situations of heavy menses or menopausal flooding, or if prone to drug dependency.

Mugwort *(Artemisia vulgaris)*
Correspondences: Southwest / Venus / Moon
Habitat: Widely found in ditches, roadsides, and scrub areas, mugwort is a plant that has spread throughout North and South America, Europe, and Asia.
Parts used: The leaves and root are used.
Plant characteristics and properties: Mugwort is an adventurer, an explorer into awareness, vigorous and positive. It is an ally of astral travel, psychic dreams, and scrying. Medicinally, mugwort supports the bladder, liver, digestion, and appetite. Useful in baths or massage oils for sore muscles, mugwort is also good for colds, flu, and in stimulating sweating or menses.
Preparation notes: Sometimes mugwort is smoked. Most commonly it is taken in infusion, 1 tablespoon 3 times a day, or in tincture, 30–60 drops as needed. Avoid excessive amounts, and do not use during pregnancy.

Mullein *(Verbascum thapsus)*
Correspondences: Southeast / Saturn / Fire
Habitat: Mullein is prolific in waste places, fields, and where soil has been disturbed.
Parts used: The leaves and flowers are used.
Plant characteristics and properties: Mullein's nature is steady but nonresistant. Its action is toward absorption and dispersal. Mullein relieves pain, irritability, and inflammation; it is best known as a respiratory healer, and also benefits the glands—it is used as a remedy for mumps. Mullein flowers are specific for earache. Its leaves are used as an astringent emollient for hemorrhoids. Mullein also helps diminish stomach cramps, dysentery, and diarrhea.
Preparation notes: Fresh mullein tincture or infusion is best.

Use 20–40 drops tincture as needed. Mullein can be taken sparingly as a smoking herb for coughs and lung illness. It is inappropriate to use in conditions of cancers or toxic swellings.

Myrrh *(Commiphora myrrha)*
Correspondences: Southwest/Moon/Water
Habitat: The trees and shrubs from which myrrh resin is taken grow in eastern Africa and Arabia.
Parts used: The resin is used.
Plant characteristics and properties: Myrrh has an aligned spiritual focus, tightknit and uplifted, making it an herb often found in ceremonies of purification or consecration. Medicinally, myrrh is an antiseptic mainly used to treat gum disease, mouth or bed sores, hemorrhoids, and sore throat. It catalyzes white blood cells. Myrrh is sometimes effective for indigestion and gas, bronchial congestion, and ulcers. It is frequently combined with frankincense in ceremonial situations.
Preparation notes: Myrrh tincture is preferred, 5–30 drops in water 4 times a day; use in smaller amounts if tinture is to be swallowed rather than used as a gargle. It can also be taken as an infusion, but not in large amounts or over a long duration. It is inappropriate with liver disease, immune disease, pregnancy, or cancer.

Nettle *(Urtica dioica* or *U. urens)*
Correspondences: Southeast/Mars
Habitat: Nettles grow almost worldwide, in forests, waste places, and damp roadsides.
Parts used: The leaves are used.
Plant characteristics and properties: Nettle celebrates vitality, active strength, and conviction. It is a mineral-rich spring blood tonic that supports the adrenals and acti-

vates digestion and circulation. Nettles can discourage hemorrhage and nosebleed; it is also an astringent for diarrhea. Tonic for hair and skin, nettle is considered an alkalizing diuretic.

Preparation notes: Use young leaves only, raw, infused, or fresh-tinctured. Tincture dosage is 15–40 drops 1 to 2 times a day.

Oatstraw *(Avena sativa)*
Correspondences: Northwest / Venus / Earth
Habitat: Oat is a widely cultivated annual grass.
Parts used: The seeds and whole plant are used.
Plant characteristics and properties: Oatstraw offers nurturance for the nurturer; it has compassion for the strong. Nutritive in nature, oatstraw, with its richness in calcium, relieves nervous exhaustion and melancholy. It is an emollient used in poultices and baths for skin disturbances; it is soothing to the bladder while tonic to muscles.

Preparation notes: Infusion or tincture are taken in small, frequent doses. The tincture dosage is 10–20 drops up to 5 times a day.

Oregon Grape *(Berberis aquifolium)*
Correspondences: West
Habitat: Oregon grape grows densely in the northwest United States.
Parts used: The root bark is used.
Plant characteristics and properties: Oregon grape has a perspective of self-acceptance. It is used for chronic skin conditions, such as eczema, psoriasis, and nonhormonal acne. Its anti-inflammatory properties make Oregon grape useful in treating arthritis. It is a digestive bitter, a remedy for low protein utilization and liver congestion.

Oregon grape also treats giardiasis and intestinal ills. It is similar to barberry but has a stronger effect on the liver and thyroid, stimulating slowly but steadily.

Preparation notes: Use small, tonic doses of tincture, 30–60 drops, or decoction, $1/2$ cup 3 times a day. Oregon grape is inappropriate in situations of pregnancy, liver disease, hyperthyroid, or acute inflammation.

Parsley (*Petroselinum sativum* or *P. crispum* or *Apium petroselinum*)

Correspondences: East/Mercury

Habitat: Parsley is usually found cultivated in gardens.

Parts used: The leaves, root, and seeds are used.

Plant characteristics and properties: Parsley focuses on threshold passage and self-respect. It is a nutrient tonic, remedy for gallstones, colitis, gastric pain, suppressed menses, and jaundice. It is a supportive herb in treating arthritis. Parsley is traditionally associated with honor and sobriety, and is used in funerals and to decorate tombs.

Preparation notes: Leaves are best used fresh, raw, or infused. Decoct the root or seeds. Tincture dose is 30–60 drops up to 4 times a day. Parsley should be avoided in pregnancy or in cases of kidney disease.

Passion Flower (*Passiflora incarnata*)

Correspondences: North/Venus/Water

Habitat: Passion flower grows wild in the southern United States and is cultivated elsewhere.

Parts used: The leaves and flowers are used.

Plant characteristics and properties: Passion flower is an ally of peaceful relationships. It is a nervine and calmative, used for hypertension, agitation, insomnia, and conflict. Passion flower helps ease nerve and shingles pain. Its antispasmodic properties make it useful for asthma.

Preparation notes: The infusion is taken 1 cup daily, or passion flower can be used as a tincture in doses of 30–60 drops up to 3 times a day. It is inappropriate in situations of bradycardia and low blood pressure, and should not be used in combination with sedative drugs. Passion flower should not be used over an extended period of time.

Pau d'Arco *(Taheebo* or *Tabebuia attissima)*
Correspondences: North
Habitat: Pau d'Arco is a tree indigenous to South America.
Parts used: The inner bark is used.
Plant characteristics and properties: Pau d'arco helps in finding relevance and coexistent balance within the web of life. Offering support to the immune system, it is antiviral and antibiotic, and assists in the abatement of tumors. Pau d'arco is specific in the treatment of skin cancer and is also used for candida. It is sometimes found in remedies for flu or colds.
Preparation notes: The decoction dose is 3 cups a day on an empty stomach. Pau d'arco can also be used in tincture form, 30–50 drops 3 times a day.

Pennyroyal *(Mentha pulegium* [European] or *Hedeoma pulegioides* [American])
Correspondences: Southwest/Mars/Fire
Habitat: Pennyroyal grows in dry fields from Minnesota to southern Quebec and Nova Scotia, and southward.
Parts used: The leaves are used.
Plant characteristics and properties: Pennyroyal's nature is to make intelligent choices and carry through clearly and without regret. Pennyroyal is an ovarian tonic; it also eases cramps and stomach disorders. Its odor repels insects and is conducive to health and alertness. Penny-

royal encourages menses. Its oil is abortifacient and can be fatal. The leaves of pennyroyal are nervine, diaphoretic, and antiseptic, used for colds, fevers, headaches, and sunstroke. Pennyroyal is a renewing wash for itching, burning skin. It is an herb associated with strength, peace, and consecration.

Preparation notes: Use an infusion, 1 cup a day, or a tincture dose of 30–60 drops 2 times a day. *The oil is for external use only; it can be fatal if used internally.* Pennyroyal should be avoided during pregnancy.

Peppermint *(Mentha piperita)*
Correspondences: Southwest/Mercury/Fire
Habitat: Peppermint thrives in moist areas ranging over much of North America.
Parts used: The leaves are used.
Plant characteristics and properties: Peppermint is an ally of acuity and rapport with context. It is a remedy for nausea, indigestion, morning and motion sickness, gas, diarrhea, cramps, and headache. It stimulates memory, reduces anxiety, and aids in restful sleep, dreams, and healing. Often used in remedies for colds, flu, and congestion, peppermint is an enlivening bath and facial herb and a tasty beverage tea.
Preparation notes: Infusion dosage is 1 cup 3 times a day, or peppermint can be taken in tincture form, 30–60 drops 3 times a day. The oil, often diluted, is used externally.

Peyote *(Anhalonium lewinii* or *A. williamsii* or *Lophophora williamsii)*
Correspondences: Southwest
Habitat: Peyote is a cactus of the southwestern and Central American deserts.
Parts used: The tops are used.

Plant characteristics and properties: Peyote's nature is
referent to higher powers. It is a visionary herb used to
attain insight and enlarge perspective beyond egoic
orientation. Peyote stimulates the heart and respiratory
systems; it is emetic and hallucinogenic, tonic in small
amounts and narcotic in large amounts. Peyote is used
medicinally to treat nervous disorders and is a hair tonic
for remedying scalp ills. Peyote is noted in its alliance to
redirection of alcoholism within the Native community.

Preparation notes: Peyote is used in water-based or powdered forms, or chewed dry. It is inappropriate for excessive or recreational use.

Pipsissewa *(Chimaphila umbellata)*
Correspondences: East
Habitat: Pipsissewa grows in northern temperate forests.
Parts used: Aerial parts are used.
Plant characteristics and properties: Pipsisssewa works
toward fluid well-being, clearing away waste matter. It is
a nonirritating diuretic for kidney and urinary ills, and
dissolves bladder stones. Pipsissewa is a lymphatic
catalyst, good for the liver, and useful in treating venereal
diseases and ulcerative eruptions.
Preparation notes: Infuse pipsissewa and take $1/2$ cup as
needed, or take in tincture, 15–40 drops up to 4 times a day.
Avoid in cases of kidney disease or anticoagulant therapy.

Plantain *(Plantago major* or *P. lanceolata, P. media)*
Correspondences: East / Venus / Earth
Habitat: Plantain is easily found in dooryards, meadows, and
roadsides almost anywhere.
Parts used: The leaves are used.
Plant characteristics and properties: Plantain has a compas-
sionate stability that finds opportunity for growth in every

situation. It is a cooling demulcent for skin inflammations, wounds, bites, burns, itches, bruises, and hemorrhoids. Plantain halts bladder bleeding and reduces profuse menses and diarrhea. It is astringent and diuretic, helpful in treating ulcers, toothaches and earaches, respiratory congestion, ringworm, and minor kidney problems.

Preparation notes: Use ¹/₂ cup raw plantain juice or pulp, or fresh infusion. Tincture dose is 10–60 drops 3 times a day.

Poke (*Phytolacca americana* or *P. decandra*)

Correspondences: Northeast / Mars / Fire

Habitat: Native to North America, poke prefers damp soils and forest verges in the eastern United States.

Parts used: The root is used.

Plant characteristics and properties: Poke likes freedom. It is associated with courage and hex-breaking. Poke remedies sore joints, rheumatism, arthritis, and congestion in the testes and uterus. It relieves lymphatic swelling and clears lymph and blood. Poke is used as a wash for scabies and fungal infections and is also effective for lingering respiratory infections and edema.

Preparation notes: Decoction is taken in 1-teaspoon doses. Poke is also used in tincture at a dose of 2–10 drops up to 3 times a day. The plant rapidly decreases in potency when dried. *Use with caution—small, short-term amounts is best.* Poke is inappropriate with pregnancy, acute inflammation, or immediately following meals. It is emetic and purgative.

Prickly Ash (*Xanthoxylum americanum* or *Zanthoxylum americanum*)

Correspondences: South / Mars / Fire

Habitat: Native to North America, this tree prefers the damp soil of the East.

Parts used: The bark and berries are used.

Plant characteristics and properties: Prickly ash participates in active integration. It improves memory and intellect and is a nervous system tonic. Prickly ash strengthens digestive fire and stimulates the lymphatic system. It aids circulation and gastric secretions and is applied to varicosities and chilblains.

Preparation notes: Use prickly ash in decoction, 2 cups daily, or in tincture form, 10–25 drops (bark) or 5–15 drops (berries) up to 3 times a day. Avoid in pregnancy or if there is active inflammation of skin, kidneys, lungs, or gastrointestinal tract.

Raspberry *(Rubus strigosus or R. idaeus)*

Correspondences: Northeast / Venus / Water

Habitat: Raspberry is an indigenous shrub growing in fields throughout North America.

Parts used: The leaves and fruit are used.

Plant characteristics and properties: Raspberry offers protective, core-strengthening nurturance. It is an excellent uterine and lymph tonic, giving context for fertility and normalizing menses. Raspberry heals wounds, ulcers, canker sores, and eye inflammation. It is a bath astringent and sore-throat gargle. Raspberry relieves nausea and cramps and increases lactation. The fruit is used to correct diarrhea; the leaves are mildly laxative.

Preparation notes: Infusion is preferred over tincture; drink 2 cups a day.

Red Clover *(Trifolium pratense)*

Correspondences: Northeast / Mercury / Air

Habitat: Red clover is abundant as a weed in fields throughout much of the United States.

Parts used: The flowers are used.

Plant characteristics and properties: Red clover believes in experiencing life's good fortune. It is nourishing and positive, an herb of fortuitousness. Red clover is a fine tonic for blood and lymph. It benefits the respiratory system, being useful for dry, irritable coughs or whooping cough. Clover soothes nerves and is a good wash for burns, ulcers, or skin eruptions. Promoting vitality in all details of living, clover encourages circulation to the capillaries.

Preparation notes: Use fresh or fresh-dried flowers in infusion or tincture, 3 times a day.

Rhubarb *(Rheum palmatum)*
Correspondences: Northwest / Venus / Earth
Habitat: This species of rhubarb is a perennial of Tibet and China.
Parts used: The root is used.
Plant characteristics and properties: Rhubarb encourages letting go of what obscures truth. It is a mild purgative for balancing yang excess, curative of constipation, diarrhea, or dysentery with gastric irritation. Rhubarb improves digestion. It is astringent, cold, and bitter.
Preparation notes: Rhubarb should be combined with buffering herbs and used sparingly. Decoction dose is 2 times a day; tincture is 15–30 drops 3 times a day. Rhubarb can also be powdered and taken in capsules. This herb is inappropriate in situations of pregnancy and acute gastrointestinal inflammation. Do not use rhubarb over an extended period of time.

Rose *(Rosa spp.)*
Correspondences: Southwest / Venus / Water
Habitat: Roses are found wild and are widely cultivated in temperate areas.
Parts used: The flowers and hips are used.
Plant characteristics and properties: Nongrasping love is rose's vision of well-being. It is an herb that refreshes and rejuvenates, calming stress and pain. Rose is a healing skin tonic for chapped hands and face and a nerve tonic for head pain and headaches from too much sun. Rose helps remedy vaginal or menstrual imbalance and is sometimes added to formulas for sore throat.
Preparation notes: Red roses are most often used, though cabbage, damask, tea, California, sweetbrier, French, and so on are also possibilities. Drink as an infusion in 1-cup doses.

Rosemary *(Rosmarinus officinalis)*
Correspondences. Southeast / Sun / Fire
Habitat: Rosemary is a Mediterranean shrub found in many gardens.
Parts used: The leaves and twigs are used.
Plant characteristics and properties: Rosemary remains true to original pattern and memory. It is associated with youth and fidelity, and the energies of winter solstice. Rosemary is a cleansing astringent and restorative; it is used for headaches, depression, and weak nerves. It promotes appetite; stimulates the liver, digestion, and circulation; and is an invigorating bath herb for invalids. Rosemary preserves the color and curl of dark hair; it discourages baldness and benefits the scalp.
Preparation notes: Infuse rosemary and take in 1-tablespoon doses, or use tincture in doses of 5–20 drops 3 times a day. Rosemary can be burned as incense to clear the air and promote healing.

Rue *(Ruta graveolens)*
Correspondences: Southwest / Mars / Fire
Habitat: Rue is native to southern Europe and northern Africa.
Parts used: The aerial parts are used.
Plant characteristics and properties: Rue encourages corrections that facilitate the transformation of karma. It is an abortifacient, nervine, emetic, and rubefaciant that activates menses and eases bowel tension and high blood pressure. It is used for expelling intestinal worms. In magical traditions, rue is considered an antidote to spells and ill wishes, heightening mental power and protection and aiding positive focus during trance.
Preparation notes: Do not take rue before meals or use in large doses. The tincture can be taken in amounts of 5–20 drops once a day, or rue can be infused and taken in dosages of $1/2$ cup daily. Use care when harvesting the leaves, which may irritate the skin, and do not boil rue. Rue is contraindicated during pregnancy.

Sage *(Salvia officinalis)*
Correspondences: Southeast / Jupiter / Air
Habitat: Sage, commonly cultivated in gardens, is native to the Mediterranean.
Parts used: The leaves are used.
Plant characteristics and properties: Sage expresses a sensible wisdom and perspective, a long-range consideration. It is an herb of longevity, an ally of menopause, a comforting bath herb for muscle aches, and an antiseptic gargle for sore throats. Sage reduces perspiration, lactation, and night sweats. It is an expectorant and relieves mild gastritis; as an external wash, sage treats itches and skin eruptions.
Preparation notes: Tincture is preferred, in a dosage of 20–30 drops up to 3 times a day. Or take a 1-cup infusion in

mouthful doses. Sage is contraindicated during pregnancy. Do not use in excess or over an extended period of time.

Sarsaparilla *(Smilax nudicaulis,* or *S. ornata, S. officinalis* or *Aralia nudicaulis)*
Correspondences: Southwest / Jupiter / Fire
Habitat: Sarsaparilla is a tropical American perennial.
Parts used: The root is used.
Plant characteristics and properties: Sarsaparilla's nature is agreeable to active engagement, to consensual movement and change. A hormone balancer (a progesterone derivative), it aids sexual vitality and testosterone activity. Sarsaparilla is a blood tonic and alterative, and a remedy for skin parasites, syphilis, rheumatism, and arthritis. Sarsaparilla works well in partnership with sassafras.
Preparation notes: Use 1–2 cups of decoction daily or 15–60 drops of tincture 3 times a day. Avoid in cases of pregnancy, steroid therapy, or gastric ulcer.

Sassafras *(Sassafras albidum* or *S. officinale)*
Correspondences: Northwest / Jupiter / Fire
Habitat: Sassafras is a tree native to the eastern half of the United States.
Parts used: The tree bark and root bark are used.
Plant characteristics and properties: Sassafras urges a positive sense of present moment. Considered a purifying herb, sassafras increases disease resistance. It is a disinfectant wash for poison ivy and oak, and for acne, eczema, psoriasis, and skin parasites. Sassafras relieves rheumatic pain and is a treatment for venereal disease. It is a supportive herb for those trying to quit smoking, and an ally associated with health and prosperity.
Preparation notes: Decoction dose for sassafras is $^1/_2$ cup

daily, or use 15–25 drops tincture 1 to 2 times a day. Do not use oil internally; in general, use sassafras with care. Avoid if there is anemia or thin blood.

Skullcap (*Scutellaria californica* or *S. laterifoilia* [preferred])
Correspondences: North / Saturn / Water
Habitat: Skullcap favors wetlands of Canada and northeast United States.
Parts used: The aerial parts are used.
Plant characteristics and properties: Skullcap offers recuperative calm. It is an herb of temperance that leaves no negative aftereffects. Skullcap is specific for convulsive disorders; it is an antispasmodic, offering assistance for cramps, epilepsy, PMS tremors, and hiccups. It is also a nervine, used to treat anxiety. Skullcap is relieving of nervous headaches, restlessness, and insomnia, and useful when coming off of narcotic drugs. Skullcap benefits the spinal cord, brain, and sympathetic nervous system, and is useful in cases of rabies and rickets.
Preparation notes: Use 20–60 drops tincture up to 3 times a day, or 1 cup of infusion 2 times a day. It is best to use fresh plants. Skullcap can also be smoked. Do not boil skullcap or combine it with sedative drugs.

Shepherd's Purse (*Capsella bursa-pastoris*)
Correspondences: Northeast
Habitat: Shepherd's purse is common to fields, roadsides, and waste places in northeastern and north central United States.
Parts used: Aerial parts are used.
Plant characteristics and properties: Shepherd's purse consolidates energy. It is an excellent hemostatic for

internal or surface bleeding; it constricts blood vessels without adversely affecting blood pressure and is high in vitamin K, which assists in blood coagulation. Shepherd's purse reduces menses and postpartum hemorrhage, promotes uterine and bowel contraction, and alleviates edema. Its astringent properties are helpful in treating diarrhea and dysentery, and its ability to reduce uric acid levels makes shepherd's purse beneficial for painful joints.

Preparation notes: Use large doses—60–90 drops—as needed for hemorrhage. For other uses the tincture dose is 20–40 drops 2 times a day, or 1 cup of infusion taken in mouthful amounts. Tincture made from fresh plants is preferred. Avoid use of shepherd's purse in pregnancy.

Slippery Elm (*Ulmus fulva*)

Correspondences: West / Saturn / Air

Habitat: Slippery elm is indigenous to areas north of the Carolinas and west of the Allegheny Mountains.

Parts used: The inner bark is used.

Plant characteristics and properties: Slippery elm has a strife-healing nature, a nourishing kindness. Its emollient and demulcent qualities soothe irritations of the gastrointestinal tract and make a comforting poultice for wounds and skin afflictions. Slippery elm is a nutritious gruel for those who are convalescing. It is a traditional remedy for coughs and tuberculosis. Other uses include application as a vermifuge for expelling worms, and a douche for leukorrhea.

Preparation notes: Mix powdered bark with water in 1:8 ratios. Simmer 10–15 minutes; use $^1/_2$ cup 3 times a day. Slippery elm can also be used in tincture form, 15–30 drops 3 times a day.

Spearmint *(Mentha viridis* or *M. spicata)*
Correspondences: Northwest / Venus / Water
Habitat: Spearmint is found in wet, temperate areas and is
    widely cultivated.
Parts used: The leaves are used.
Plant characteristics and properties: Spearmint's nature is
    intelligently compassionate. It is an herb associated with
    love and with mental power. Medicinally, spearmint is
    used to benefit kidneys and bladder, and as a remedy for
    fever, sore throat, morning sickness, and vomiting. It is
    similar to peppermint but not as pungent or stimulating.
Preparation notes: Use an infusion or tincture as needed.

Spikenard *(Aralia racemosa* or *A. nudicaulis)*
Correspondences: Southwest / Venus / Water
Habitat: Spikenard prefers rich forest areas of the eastern
    United States
Parts used: The root is used.
Plant characteristics and properties: Spikenard's nature is to
    transfer and transform. It facilitates childbirth; it is also
    used for chronic coughs and asthma. Spikenard is dia-
    phoretic and expectorant. It can be applied as a poultice
    to swellings, or taken as a remedy for cystitis.
Preparation notes: 1–2 cups is the dose for decoction, or take
    10–30 drops tincture. Avoid spikenard during pregnancy.

Squawvine *(Mitchella repens)* aka Partridgeberry
Correspondences: North
Habitat: Squawvine grows around the bases of trees and
    stumps in eastern forests of the United States and
    Canada.
Parts used: Aerial parts are used.
Plant characteristics and properties: Squawvine is an herb of
    basic, grounded resiliency. As a uterine tonic it strength-

ens uterine lining and function, and prepares the uterus for birth in the final six weeks of pregnancy. Mineral-rich squawvine also tones the prostate, and is remedial for painful, scant menses. It is an astringent useful as a skin and eye wash and in treating colitis.

Preparation notes: The infusion dose is 1 cup 3 times a day, or squawvine can be taken in tincture form, 30–90 drops up to 3 times a day. It is inappropriate during the first two trimesters of pregnancy.

St. Johnswort *(Hypericum perforatum)*

Correspondences: Northeast/Sun/Fire

Habitat: In the eastern and far western parts of the United States, St. Johnswort is prolific in sunny fields and grows in dry, gravely soils.

Parts used: The flowers and aerial parts are used.

Plant characteristics and properties: St. Johnswort urges a healing happiness, a sensitivity able to interact with life. It is an anti-inflammatory nerve tonic for insomnia, depression, sciatica, spinal shock or injury, and nerve injuries in the extremities. St. Johnswort eases menopausal irritability and is a preventive for tetanus. The flowers are used for earache, sunburn, bruises, aches, wounds, swellings, varicosities, jaundice, anemia, and nerve damage. St. Johnswort is associated with the energies of Midsummer's eve, and with protection against fire, thunder, and evil.

Preparation notes: Use fresh leaves as an infusion, up to 1 cup daily, or use tincture form, 10–30 drops up to 3 times a day. St. Johnswort is often used in homeopathic form. Flowers are infused in oil for external applications. The use of St. Johnswort can cause photosensitivity.

Strawberry *(Fragaria vesca)*
Correspondences: Southwest/Venus/Water
Habitat: Strawberry is a plant found wild in forest clearings and fields in Canada and in the northern United States south to Virginia and Missouri. It is also widely cultivated in gardens.
Parts used: The leaves and fruit are used.
Plant characteristics and properties: Strawberry's perspective is of nurturant pleasure. It is an astringent for oily skin; strawberry leaves are nutritive, and the juice of the berries is a sunburn remedy. Strawberry reduces fever, gout, diarrhea, and morning sickness.
Preparation notes: Use 2 tablespoons of juice daily, or 5–15 drops 3 times a day of leaf tincture. The infusion dose is $^1/_2$ cup 3 times a day.

Tansy *(Tanacetum vulgare)*
Correspondences: Southwest/Venus/Water
Habitat: Tansy thrives on roadsides and around house foundations in Europe and the northern United States.
Parts used: The aerial parts are used.
Plant characteristics and properties: Tansy banishes what is unwanted; it is an ally of release. The seeds are used as a vermifuge. The leaves and flowers repel moths, ants, and flies, and are abortant and nervine. Tansy is considered an antidote to black magic. Hot infusions increase circulation. Tansy is also applied as a bitter digestive, a skin wash, and a salve for bruises.
Preparation notes: Tansy is taken in small doses for short durations: *It is considered poisonous in doses over 15–20 drops of tincture, or when used longer than seven to ten days.* Avoid tansy during pregnancy.

Thyme *(Thymus vulgaris)*
Correspondences: Southwest / Venus / Water
Habitat: Thyme is native to southern Europe but is widely
cultivated in the United States.
Parts used: The aerial parts are used.
Plant characteristics and properties: Thyme has a vigorous
patience. It is an ally of courage, psychic strength, consecration, and release of regrets. Medicinally, thyme is a
carminative and expectorant for whooping cough and
bronchitis. It has an antiseptic effect on wounds and
fungus infections, and stimulates circulation and digestion. Thyme can be smoked to counteract headache and
drowsiness, or burned as a purifying incense.
Preparation notes: Fresh plant material is preferred for
tincture; the tincture dose is 10–20 drops 3 times a day.
One cup of infusion can be taken in small, frequent doses,
or thyme can be used externally in oil form. Avoid excessive use—thyme can overstimulate the thyroid.

Unicorn Root *(Aletris farinosa)* aka Colicroot, Stargrass
Correspondences: Southeast
Habitat: Fields and forest borders in the Great Lakes states,
Maine, and parts of Ontario are where to look for this
herb.
Parts used: The root is used.
Plant characteristics and properties: Unicorn root has the
integrity of innocence. Its traditional use is to ward off
evil. Unicorn root tones digestion and prompts appetite;
it is helpful for anorexia, and relieves colic and gas. The
reproductive system derives some benefit from use of
unicorn root.
Preparation notes: Use dried root only; decoction dosage is 3
times a day, or tincture is taken before meals at a dose of
30–60 drops.

Uva Ursi *(Arctostaphylos uva-ursi)* aka Bearberry
Correspondences: Southeast / Mars
Habitat: Uva ursi likes sandy soils. It grows in both the
northern United States and Europe.
Parts used: The leaves are used.
Plant characteristics and properties: Uva ursi facilitates
access to deeper spiritual resource. It is a remedial bladder tonic for treating cystitis and bedwetting. As an
astringent it tones the bladder walls and is helpful as a
douche or sitzbath for infections, hemorrhoids, or postpartum healing. Uva ursi is smoked or burned as incense
for astral or psychic work or to invoke prophecy. Other
medicinal uses are for bronchitis, Bright's disease, and
gonorrhea.
Preparation notes: The tincture dose for uva ursi is 10–40
drops up to 4 times a day, or a hot infusion can be taken
in small, frequent doses. Uva ursi should not be used
over extended periods or during pregnancy. Do not take
this herb in conjunction with anticoagulants.

Valerian *(Valeriana officinalis)*
Correspondences: Northwest / Venus / Water
Habitat: Valerian is common to Europe and can be found in
scrub areas of the northeastern United States as a naturalized import.
Parts used: The root is used.
Plant characteristics and properties: Valerian offers respite,
truce, moratorium. It has a strong sedative effect on pain
and headache associated with tension, and on nerve
disorders, insomnia, sleeplessness due to caffeine, epilepsy,
and restless low fevers. Valerian relaxes the heart muscle; it
is antihypoxic and reduces aggression and hysteria.
Preparation notes: The root's odor increases as it loses potency; fresh root is best. Do not boil valerian. Use small,
frequent amounts—30–40 drops of tincture up to 3 times

a day, or mouthful doses of infusion. Do not use valerian during pregnancy, in the case of inflammations, or for extended periods—its effect can become depressive or counterproductive.

Vervain *(Verbena officinalis* or *V. hastata)* (Note: This is not the same plant as lemon verbena.)
Correspondences: Southwest / Venus / Earth
Habitat: Often found on riversides, blue vervain, a naturalized import, grows in North America from New York southward.
Parts used: The aerial parts are used.
Plant characteristics and properties: Vervain teaches about faith and letting go of bitterness. It has ancient associations with druidic magic and European pagan traditions. A nervine, vervain calms hyperactivity, irritability, and headaches. Taken warm, it is useful for fevers, colds, and viral infections. It is a poulticing herb for head and nerve pain, or for rheumatism.
Preparation notes: Use $1/2$ cup of infusion or 25–40 drops of tincture as needed. Vervain is inappropriate in situations of pregnancy, liver disease, low blood pressure, or sedative drugs.

Violet *(Viola odorata* or *V. papilionacea)*
Correspondences: Northwest / Venus / Water
Habitat: Of European origin, violets now grow wild in fields and forest borders. The common blue violet is found in North Dakota, Quebec, and southward from Maine.
Parts used: The leaves and flowers are used.
Plant characteristics and properties: Violet's nature emanates beauty, love, and luck. It moderates anger, eases the heart, sweetens sleep, and is associated with peace, simplicity, sexual joy, and the Little People. Violet is a

remedial wash or lotion for the complexion; its leaves are used in treatment of cancer, cysts, and lymph ills. Violet is rich in vitamin C. It is a good children's laxative and also relieves dizziness, coughs, and colds.

Preparation notes: Infusion is the preferred form for using violet leaves.

White Oak *(Quercus alba)*

Correspondences: South/Sun

Habitat: White oak is a tree native to North America, mainly growing in the eastern half of the United States.

Parts used: The inner bark is used.

Plant characteristics and properties: The gather and focus of will is embodied in oak. It is a powerful astringent that halts bleeding, strengthens capillaries, and remedies hemorrhoids, varicosities, mouth and gum sores, gastritis, and ulcers. White oak is used as a vaginal douche and also benefits the spleen. Acorns are grated to treat diarrhea.

Preparation notes: Use a decoction in ¹/₂-cup doses, or tincture, 30–60 drops, as needed.

White Willow *(Salix alba)*

Correspondences: West/Moon/Water

Habitat: Native to moist places of Europe, Africa, and Asia, white willow now also grows in the northeastern United States.

Parts used: The inner bark is used.

Plant characteristics and properties: Willow's perspective is of flexible connections, the interwoven strands of life. It is a tree of mystery, associated with divination and love. White willow is used to treat pain and headaches. It is an astringent disinfectant for wounds and inflammations, and it discourages internal bleeding.

Preparation notes: Use white willow in cold decoction, 1 cup daily in mouthful doses, or take in tincture form, 15–60 drops 2 to 3 times a day.

Wild Cherry *(Prunus avium* or *P. serotina, P. virginiana)*
Correspondences: Southwest / Venus
Habitat: This tree grows in the eastern half of the United States. *Prunus virginiana* also grows in the northern United States and in southern Canada.
Parts used: The inner bark is used.
Plant characteristics and properties: Wild cherry sees well-being in terms of open passages. It eases childbirth pain and clears breathing passages during dry, hot, bronchial coughing. Wild cherry also clears eye inflammations and is a digestive tonic.
Preparation notes: Cold infuse and drink 3 times a day, or use a tincture, 30–90 drops up to 4 times a day. Wild cherry is inappropriate in cases of low blood pressure, or cardiovascular or respiratory depression.

Wild Lettuce *(Lactuca virosa* or *L. canadensis)*
Correspondences: North
Habitat: Wild lettuce grows easily in poor and disturbed soils. It is a naturalized import.
Parts used: The leaves are used.
Plant characteristics and properties: Wild lettuce offers attention to and detachment from compulsion. It is a sedative and hypnotic for release from agitation, insomnia, hyperactivity, and pain. Wild lettuce diminishes cramps, coughs, and colic.
Preparation notes: Wild lettuce is used in infusion or tincture. Because of its strong alkaloid properties, it is important to exercise caution in using this herb.

Wild Yam *(Dioscorea villosa)*
Correspondences: West
Habitat: Wild yam is a perennial of the eastern United States found in thickets and ledges.
Parts used: The root is used.
Plant characteristics and properties: It is wild yam's nature to perceive and respond to situations before they reach crisis, restoring balance. Wild yam is a steroid precursor for glandular normalizing. It helps prevent miscarriage and may be useful during menopause. It calms the nerves; its antispasmodic action is helpful for morning sickness, colic, colitis, and ovarian pain. Wild yam also aids the gall bladder and uterus, and is applied to the treatment of rheumatoid arthritis.
Preparation notes: Take mouthful doses of infusion, or 20–50 drops of tincture up to 4 times a day. Use with care—wild yam's influence on hormonal balances may, with long-term use, have adverse effecs on other aspects of well-being.

Wintergreen *(Gaultheria procumbens)*
Correspondences: West/Moon/Water
Habitat: Wintergreen is an evergreen shrub of North American forests and clearings.
Parts used: The leaves are used.
Plant characteristics and properties: Wintergreen reestablishes fundamental flow patterns. It heals chronic mucus discharge and rheumatic inflammation, and is an excellent liniment for muscular and skeletal problems. Wintergreen is diuretic and astringent but increases menses and lactation. It is traditionally associated with protection and hex-breaking.
Preparation notes: Use 1 cup of infusion a day, in mouthful doses, or 5–15 drops of tincture 1 to 2 times a day. The essential oil of wintergreen can be irritating to the skin.

Witch Hazel *(Hamamelis virginiana)*
Correspondences: East/Sun/Fire
Habitat: Witch hazel is a small tree growing in moist forests in eastern North America.
Parts used: The leaves and bark are used.
Plant characteristics and properties: Witch hazel is concerned with reconciliation. It is a highly astringent herb, tonic to uterus and vagina and relieving of pelvic congestion, bruises, and varicosities. Witch hazel alleviates hemorrhoids, dysentery, poison ivy, bites and stings, sunburn, and eye inflammations. It is used to control bleeding, and is often the wood of choice for divining rods.
Preparation notes: Dosage for witch hazel is 1 cup daily of infusion, in mouthful doses, or 20–60 drops of tincture up to 3 times a day.

Wormwood *(Artemisia absinthium)*
Correspondences: Southwest/Mars/Fire
Habitat: Wormwood, a European native, now thrives on North American roadsides and waste places.
Parts used: Aerial parts are used.
Plant characteristics and properties: Wormwood suggests taking risks to invoke peace. It is a remedial vermifuge and insect repellent, a strong liver and stomach herb, and antiseptic. Wormwood is magically used for scrying, dreamwork, and protection.
Preparation notes: Take wormwood in small doses only: 8–10 drops of tincture up to 3 times a day, or ½ cup of infusion per day in teaspoon amounts. Use care when harvesting the leaves, which can irritate the skin.

Yarrow *(Achillea millefolium* or *A. lanulosa)*
Correspondences: Southwest / Venus / Water
Habitat: Yarrow is found all over the world in poor soil, fields, and roadsides.
Parts used: The aerial parts are used.
Plant characteristics and properties: Yarrow has an intrepid nature—it is interactive and supportive. Yarrow relieves fever, including typhoid, and breaks up colds and flu. Yarrow is excellent for urinary ills, and can be employed as a douche for leukorrhea. It reduces bleeding, lowers blood pressure, encourages appetite, and treats measles and other eruptive ills. Yarrow is traditionally associated with divination and the I Ching.
Preparation notes: The tincture dose for yarrow is 10–40 drops 4 times a day; the infusion dose is 3 cups daily. Yarrow needs to be steeped only briefly. It is inappropriate in situations of pregnancy, bradycardia, coagulation problems, or kidney disease.

Yellow Dock *(Rumex crispus)*
Correspondences: Northeast
Habitat: Yellow dock is a weed of the fields of Europe and north central and northeastern United States.
Parts used: The root is used.
Plant characteristics and properties: Yellow dock's perspective is grounded and vigorous, a harmonious integration of mind and body. An iron-rich blood tonic, yellow dock is specific for chronic, dry, sluggish skin conditions and for constipation caused by insufficient metabolism of fat. Yellow dock is also a beneficial ally for the liver.
Preparation notes: The decoction dose for yellow dock is 1–2 cups daily, or 10–40 drops tincture up to 2 times a day. Excessive amounts of yellow dock are cathartic and irritating. Do not use the plant raw; yellow dock is particularly good tinctured in apple cider vinegar.

Yerba Mansa *(Anemiopsis californica)*
Correspondences: East
Habitat: Yerba mansa is a plant of Central America.
Parts used: The leaves are used.
Plant characteristics and properties: Yerba mansa attends to the details and balances of good relationship. It heals mucous membranes, eases colitis and stomach ulcers, and is healing to sinus infections, gum inflammations, cystitis, and joint inflammations. Antiseptic and astringent, yerba mansa is useful whenever there is excess secretion, and also brings balance to acidic urine.
Preparation notes: Use yerba mansa in infusion or tincture doses of 20–60 drops up to 4 times a day.

Yerba Santa *(Eriodictyon californicum)*
Correspondences: South
Habitat: Yerba santa is native to the dry rocky areas of Oregon and California.
Parts used: The leaves are used.
Plant characteristics and properties: Yerba santa believes in the power of beauty as an element of healing and awareness. Medicinally, yerba santa is a blood tonic and an expectorant for bronchial coughs, asthma, and sinus congestion. Externally, it is used as a poultice for sprains and bruises.
Preparation notes: The dose for yerba santa is 20–30 drops of tincture up to 4 times a day or 1–2 cups of infusion taken in mouthful doses. This herb can be smoked for asthma.

APPENDICES

General Tips for Growing Common Garden Herbs

Angelica
Biennial, 4'.
Sow outside in midsummer or fall in moist, light, well-drained, medium-rich soil. Needs partial shade. Angelica self-seeds, but is difficult to germinate. Lovely spring flowers.

Anise
Annual 2'.
Sow outside—anise does not transplant well. Needs full sun, light soil, generous watering. Best to use fresh seeds each year.

Basil
Annual, 18".
Sow indoors in spring. Basil likes rich, sandy soil. Water regularly. Good companion plant to tomatoes. Can be grown in pots.

Bergamot
Perennial, 18-36".
Propagate by root division—divide every three years and reset. Grows in moist soils in open spaces. Attracts bees.

Borage
Annual, 30".
Sow from spring to fall. Reseeds itself. Borage is drought-resistant—it tolerates poor soil but prefers rich. Improves growth of other plants, especially tomatoes, strawberries, and squash. Beautiful blue flowers. Attracts bees.

Calendula
Annual, 2'.
Sow indoors in spring. Needs full sun, ample water. Calendula is easy to grow, and has wonderful bright blooms. Good companion to potatoes, beans, and strawberries.

Catnip
Perennial, 18".
Sow indoors or use root divisions. Catnip self-seeds. Grows in dry, sandy soil in full sun. If your cats get a whiff of it, you may lose your catnip.

Chamomile, German
Annual, 18".
Sow indoors. Needs dry, light soil and full sun. German chamomile is drought-tolerant.

Chamomile, Roman
Perennial, 6".
Sow indoors. Roman chamomile self-seeds. Needs average soil, not too much shade. A very hardy plant.

Chives
Perennial, 1'.
Sow indoors in early spring, in rich soil. Easily grown—can be put in pots. Needs full sun. Helps repel aphids and is a good companion to carrots and lettuce.

Comfrey
Perennial, 3'.
Plant by root division in early spring, in rich, moist soil. Propagates enthusiastically. Needs full sun or partial shade.

Costmary
Perennial, 3'.
Use root divisions; sow in dry, medium-fertile soil. Needs sun in order to blossom.

Echinacea
Perennial, 2'.
Start indoors by root division. Seeds need sixty-day stratification at 41 degrees. Average soil is fine. Dappled afternoon shade is ideal, with well-drained soil and generous watering. Keep well weeded.

Fennel
Annual, 30".
Sow outdoors in well-limed soil. Set apart from other plants. Likes sunshine.

Fenugreek
Annual, 18".
Sow indoors in rich soil and full sun.

Feverfew
Perennial, 3'.
Early spring sowing or root division. May not remain perennial if winter soil is too wet, or if it is allowed to go to seed. Tolerates dry soil. Has pretty flowers.

Horehound
Perennial, 18".
Sow indoors or use root divisions. Horehound self-seeds. Needs hot, dry, chalky, light soil in sun or partial shade.

Hyssop
Perennial, 2'.
Start indoors. Likes well-limed, sandy soil. Needs full sun or partial shade. Keep away from radishes or dandelions, but partner with grapes. Attracts bees.

Lady's mantle
Perennial, 1'.
Propagate by root divisions. Lady's mantle self-seeds. Prefers rich, moist soil; needs full sun.

Lavender
Perennial, 2–3'.
Start indoors or propagate by stem cuttings, root division, or layering. Grow in light, limed soil, in full sun. The seeds are slow to germinate. Appreciates winter protection. Wonderful flowers.

Lemon balm
Perennial 2'.
Sow after last frost in medium-dry, light, sandy soil, or use root divisions. Needs sun or partial shade. Lemon balm self-seeds and tends to spread. Attracts bees.

Lemon verbena
Tender perennial, 3'.
Grow from stem cuttings. Likes rich soil. Smells wonderful.

Lovage
Perennial, 6".
Sow indoors or out. Likes moist, rich soil. Full sun or partial shade. Easy to grow but will winterkill in cold climes.

Mints
Perennial, heights vary.
Grow in rich, moist soils. Generally propagate by root divisions. Can withstand full sun but prefers partial shade. Spreads easily.

Oregano
Perennial, 2'.
Propagate by root divisions. Likes rich, chalky, dry soil and full sun. Attracts bees.

Parsley
Biennial, 1'.
Sow outdoors in rich soil. Needs sun or partial shade. The best harvest is in its first year.

Pennyroyal
Perennial, 1'.
Start indoors or sow in warm soil. Grows well in moist clay soil. Pennyroyal is slow to germinate. Likes partial shade—will die back in dry weather. Creeps. Appreciates compost. Repels bugs.

Rosemary
Tender perennial, 2'.
Propagate with stem cuttings—slow to germinate from seed. Needs well-drained, alkaline soil and full sun. Loves to be misted. Needs winter cover. Attracts bees, repels bugs. Companion to carrots but not to tomatoes or potatoes. Rosemary is drought-tolerant.

Rue
Perennial, 2'.
Start indoors or by root division. Grows easily—likes sun but tolerates partial shade. Repels flies. Do not grow near cabbage, broccoli, sage, or basil. Pretty, blue-green foliage.

Sage, garden
Perennial, 2'.
Sow indoors, use stem cuttings, or divide roots. Likes well-limed, sandy, well-drained soil and full sun. Deters insects. Companion to carrots.

Southernwood
Perennial, 3'.
Propagate through root division, cuttings, or layering. Needs winter protection. Grows in average soil and full sun.

Sweet woodruff
Perennial, 10".
Propagate from root divisions or stem cuttings. Needs shade and a leafy, well-drained, moist soil that is loose and porous.

Tansy
Perennial, 3'.
Use root divisions. Grows in average soil, full sun. Can be invasive. Tansy repels insects. Has fern-like foliage and yellow button flowers.

Wormwood
Perennial, 3'.
Sow indoors or grow from root division. Prefers sun but tolerates partial shade. Grows in average, moist soil. Repels insects. Keep away from fennel, sage, caraway, anise, and all seedlings and young plants.

Yarrow
Perennial, 2'.
Grow from root divisions in moderately rich, somewhat moist soil, in full sun. Tolerates drought. Increases the aroma and medicinal potency of aromatic herbs grown near it.

Forms for Medicinal Application of Herbs

The following are some of the forms traditionally chosen for applying medicinal herbs. Containers or heating vessels for plants are usually glass, stone, or steel, and the use of an open flame is preferable to electric heat.

Juice
Juice is made by crushing fresh herbs and straining the pulp through cloth. Many nutrient herbs are used in this form.

Poultice
Fresh herbs are macerated, grated, or pulped and directly applied to the body for treating stings, bites, splinters, swellings, lacerations, and fractures.

Paste
Herbs are ground and mixed with a small amount of water. Sometimes honey, ghee, or oil is added. Paste can be used externally or internally.

Plaster
Cloth is thinly spread with honey and sprinkled with powdered herbs. It is fastened directly to the affected part of the body to ease congestion or pain.

Compress
A stew made with herbs and hot water is wrapped in a cloth

and applied to aches, sprains, strains, congestion, cysts, and inflammations.

Fomentation
A cloth is soaked in herbal infusion or decoction and applied as hot as possible to the body.

Hot infusion
One ounce of dried or 2 ounces of fresh leaves or flowers are combined with 1 pint to 1 quart boiling water, covered, and steeped for 10 minutes to 4 hours, depending on the herb, then strained and used. Seeds, berries, and hips generally steep for 15 to 30 minutes.

Cold infusion
Herbs steep, covered, in cool water for 1 to 2 hours. This method is used for powdered herbs, plants with volatile oils, and herbs like wild cherry whose medicinal qualities are marred by heat.

Decoction
One ounce of roots or bark are simmered, covered, for 20 to 30 minutes in 1 pint of water, or are steeped for 8 hours, then strained. Concentrated decoctions are made by first simmering the herbs, then uncovering and allowing evaporation on a flame low enough that the mixture steams without simmering. This process is complete when half the original fluid is gone.

Tincture
An extract is made by soaking 1 to 4 ounces of fresh herbs (or sometimes dried herbs) in 8 to 12 ounces of 60- to 100-proof alcohol. The covered mixture stands for 2 to 6 weeks, and can be periodically shaken or stirred. The plant material is then strained out and pressed. The extraction process is best initiated at new moon and finished on a full moon. Tinctures are also made with apple cider vinegar or glycerin instead of alcohol, though this sometimes changes what properties are extracted. Tinctures are used in small doses, internally or externally.

Alchemy tincture

An extract is made, then the strained plant material is calcined to a fine ash, powdered, and added back into the liquid. This combination is redistilled. Details for making alchemy tinctures can be found in Frater Albertus's *Alchemist's Handbook.*

Liniment

Using isopropyl alcohol as the base, a tincture is made for the purpose of rubbing onto sprains, strains, contusions, aches, and painful joints. A liniment is for external use only.

Syrup

Add ½ cup of honey to a pint of strained, hot, concentrated decoction, or boil 3 tablespoons of raw sugar in 1 pint of decoction. Use for sore throats and coughs.

Oil

Use olive, sesame, coconut, or safflower oil as an infusion medium. (Sweet almond, grape seed, apricot kernel, avocado, and wheat germ oils are often used as bases or additions for massage oils.) Crush herbs and cover with oil. Let stand for 1 to 7 days. Strain, press, and bottle. Tinctures or essential oils can be added. Medicinal oils are used externally for massage and for treating burns, cuts, rashes, aches, strains, growths, swelling, stings, and so on. They should not be used on puncture wounds or inflamed areas where air circulation is needed. Ayurvedic oils are made by decocting 1 part herb, 16 parts water, and 4 parts oil, simmering until all the water evaporates.

Salve and ointment

Add 1 tablespoon grated beeswax to 1 ounce of decocted or infused herbal oil and gently heat until wax dissolves. Salves use more wax than ointments, to make a firmer consistency. Essential oils can be added immediately before the salve or ointment is poured into a jar. One to 3 drops of benzoin tincture per 1 ounce of oil can be added, as a preservative.

Bath
Make 2 quarts of infusion or decoction, strain, and add to your bathwater. Baths are used as comforting, relaxing mediums, and for treating aches, cuts, rashes, abrasions, and congestion. For a sitzbath, use a basin large enough to sit in. A footbath is useful for administering remedies to children, for drawing out toxicities, or for drawing in the heat of warming herbs. A vapor bath can be administered as either a general room humidifier or a concentrated treatment. To concentrate the vapors, make a tent with a towel and position the upper body over a bowl or pan of gently steaming infusion or decoction. Do not do this over a stove, or position the face too close to the steam. This treatment is used for tonifying skin; treating colds, coughs, congestion, sinus problems, and bronchitis; and for drawing out splinters.

Smoke
Some throat, sinus, or lung ailments are eased by inhaling smoke from smoldering herbs. This technique should not be overused.

Powder
Dried herbs are ground and the powders encapsulated. These are effective for gastrointestinal disorders. With some exceptions, powders only retain potency for one to three months,

Pill
Water or honey is added to powdered herbs and rolled into pellets. These are best taken with warm water. Pills are used for convenience or to avoid the strong taste of certain herbs.

Pillow and sachet
Fragrant herbs can be tucked into small pillows or natural cloth pouches. These are used to scent spaces such as closets and drawers, as insect deterrents, as dream inducers, or as calming devices. Orris root is often added to extend the duration of the sachet's fragrance.

Essential oil
These oils are most often made through steam distilling—this is generally not a home project. Essential oils are extremely concentrated; they are used externally (and, with some oils, internally) in minute or diluted amounts. They are often added to medicinal oils and salves, and to shampoos, perfumes, soaps, potpourris, candles, and toothpastes.

Plant Associations Within the Web of Life

Practioners of shamanic or spiritual healing have traditionally applied to their work specific correspondences among various inhabitants of the web of life. Altar configurations, in arrangements both simple and elaborate, usually demonstrate such systems of correspondence, such as in using certain plants to signify the cardinal directions. Medicine bundles also generally contain a collection of charged representative objects or plant materials whose energies are associated with certain purposes. These representative objects give the altar or bundle its particular focus or emphasis as well as its harmonious connectedness to the larger cosmos. The community of energies present on an altar or in a medicine bundle is a spiritual ecosystem, a charged, inhabited context in which specific resonances are invoked, housed, expressed, and strengthened.

Knowledge, belief, intention, and procedure play important roles in the application of correspondences; it should be respectfully remembered that objects such as claws, feathers, teeth, or figurines, or rocks and plant material also manifest resonant realities without our understanding or interaction. The practical use of correspondences pertaining to the Directions of the medicine wheel or attributed to totems, or within systems such as astrology, alchemy, Kabbalism, and so forth, is a potent way of expanding awareness of relationship. That awareness can then be a tool of healing.

For the shamanic practitioner, healing is a realization of interconnection and a reiteration of wholeness. Use of correspondences weaves the strands of manifested life, mirrored in a coherence in awareness, so that what seemed fragmented becomes integrated. This shift in perception resonates through other stratas of experience, catalyzing healing both personal and transpersonal, physical and psychological. Sacred work with correspondences repeats a creation pattern aligning the practitioner with wholeness.

Medicine Wheel Correlations for Herbs

The following list groups herbs by directional orientation. This orientation is not geographical, but is instead a way of viewing the spiritual natures as well as the healing medicines of plants.

Each Direction indicates a precinct of specific energies, an aspect of wholeness. This listing includes cross-quarter groupings as well as cardinal Directions to make an eight-pointed medicine wheel. The Southeast combines the airy nature of the East with the fiery energies of the South, as the Southwest carries the Fire into the realm of Water. The Northwest joins Water and Earth, and the Northeast brings Earth to Air. These elemental groupings may also relate to systems of herb energetics as used in Chinese and Ayurvedic medicine. Such systems aid the practitioner in choosing appropriate remedies for different situations, and can be applied to ceremonial or spiritual work as well.

East—Corresponding to Air

Blackberry
Black cohosh
Buchu
Cleavers
Coltsfoot
Coriander
Couchgrass
Daisy
Dandelion
Eyebright
Fern
Gravel root
Hydrangea
Kava-kava
Lady's mantle
Lavender
Lungwort
Meadowsweet
Mistletoe
Parsley
Pipsissewa
Plantain
Pumpkin seeds
Red root
Rose hips
Tobacco
Watercress
Wild carrot
Witch hazel
Yerba mansa
Yucca

Southeast—Corresponding to Air and Fire

Angelica
Agrimony
Anise
Basil
Beth root
Calendula
Caraway
Cardamom
Chamomile
Chicory
Costmary
Dill
Ephedra
Frankincense
Ginseng
Horehound
Hyssop
Lovage
Marjoram
Mullein
Nettles
Oregano
Osha
Rosemary
Sage (garden)
Sunflower
Uva ursi

South—Corresponding to Fire

Black pepper
Bloodroot
Cayenne
Cinnamon
Cloves
Copal

Galangal
Garlic
Ginger
Grindelia
Yerba santa

Southwest—Corresponding to Fire and Water

Bayberry
Blue cohosh
Boneset
Catnip
Chaste tree
Cinquefoil
Cotton root
Corn silk
Cubeb
Damiana
Elder flowers
False unicorn
Feverfew
Horsetail
Lemon balm
Mugwort

Myrrh
Pennyroyal
Peppermint
Pleurisy root
Prairie sage
Rose
Rue
Sarsaparilla
Saw palmetto
Spikenard
Tansy
Thyme
Vervain
Wormwood
Yarrow
Yohimbe

West—Corresponding to Water

Aconite
Belladonna
Bitterroot
Calamus
Comfrey root
Datura
Devil's club
Dittany of Crete
Dong qui
Gotu kola
Irish moss
Linseed
Lobelia
Marshmallow
Motherwort
Nightblooming cereus
Oregon grape
Peony root
Psyllium
Slippery elm
Solomon's seal
Tiger lily
Wild yam
Wintergreen

Northwest—Corresponding to Water and Earth

Aloe
Blessed thistle
Borage
Bugleweed
Burdock
Cascara sagrada
Chickweed
Comfrey leaves
Fenugreek
Henbane
Hibiscus
Jewelweed
Kelp
Licorice
Rhubarb root
Senna
Stillingia
Valerian
Violet

North—Corresponding to Earth

Alfalfa
Bittersweet
Hops
Lady's slipper
Pansy
Passion flower
Skullcap
Self-heal
Southernwood
Sweetgrass
Wood betony

Northeast—Corresponding to Earth and Air

Barberry	Honeysuckle
Blue flag	Northeast mandrake
Centaury	Milk thistle
Chaparral	Poke
Culver's root	Purslane
Dandelion root	Raspberry leaves
Echinacea	Red clover
Elecampane	Scotch broom
Gentian	Shepherd's purse
Goldenseal	St. Johnswort
Greater celandine	Yellow dock

Medicine Wheel Correlations for Trees

Trees can also be grouped by their affiliations with the Directions on the medicine wheel. Trees related to the East are those of awakening and focus. The mental energies of the East are devoted to thought, inspiration, and clarity of discernment. Trees placed in the South relate to the fiery vitality that promotes action, movement, and lively relationship. Creative sexuality is also an energy of the South, represented by many of the trees within the South grouping. West is the direction of introspection, dreaming, ceremony, and mystery. Often the West's trees grow beside water and convey those fluid qualities of reflection and emotional depth. Their medicines may be ones that affect fluid balances in the body or influence the heart and circulation. In the North direction is stability, continuity, age, and renewal. Trees in this grouping often live to be ancient giants, or emanate energies of protection and healing. North medicine is enduring and encompassing.

The partnering of trees with sacred Directions can be applied to the arrangement of ceremonial sites, or used as an aspect of ceremony. The perspective of medicine wheel correspondences can also be incorporated into your understanding and use of bark, fruit, and other of trees' gifts for healing. Directional categorization may help in devising balanced remedies, or may give additional resource for the making of medicine bundles.

East—Corresponding to Air

Beech	Olive
Hawthorne	Pine
Hazel	Sandalwood
Hickory	Sycamore
Linden	Tulip tree
Maple	

South—Corresponding to Fire

Alder	Locust
Bay	Magnolia
Cedar	Mulberry
Cherry	Oak
Dogwood	Prickly ash
Eucalyptus	Sassafras
Juniper	

West—Corresponding to Water

Apple	Fringetree
Ash	Hemlock
Aspen	Larch
Black haw	Madrone
Buckthorn	Poplar
Butternut	Willow
Cottonwood	Witch hazel
Cypress	

North—Corresponding to Earth

Birch	Rowan
Elm	Serviceberry
Fir	Sequoia
Holly	Spruce
Horse chestnut	Walnut
Palm	Yew
Redwood	

Herb/Animal Correlations

There are several levels on which herb/animal correspondences operate. Interrelationship is often expressed through the tendency to compare a plant's visible characteristics to those of an animal. This is easily seen in common names used for many herbs. Something about the herb—leaf texture, shape, and so on—evokes the image of an animal, which can then be used in work with totem energies as relationships that can be translated into spiritual resonances. Another level is that of traditional associations between certain plants and animals based on more subtle or esoteric relationships. For example, horehound could be used in conjunction with dog medicine due to the evocative inclusion of the word hound in the plant's name, or it could be used in relation to bull energies because, in Kabbalistic tradition, horehound is associated with Horus, the bull-headed deity form.

A third level of correspondence is that of significant physical interaction between a plant and animal. Henbane and wolfbane are so named because of their association with poisoning certain animals; catnip is a favorite herb for feline enjoyment. It makes no difference which levels of association you operate on as long as you have a definite sense of relationship between the herb and the animal you are working with. It could be an association altogether personal, such as making a dog medicine bundle with leaves from a bush your dog always beds down under, regardless of whether or not the plant is generally linked with dogs. The importance is in your clear sense of relationship between the two, and the pattern of association demonstrated.

An animal ally might suggest certain plant correspondences to you, or a plant totem may reveal its animal correlates in the course of your work together. This, the most direct means of discerning correspondences, may sometimes yield the most idiosyncratic results. Herb/animal partnerships can be an aspect of ongoing spiritual work with totems and allies or it may be situational. It is work with resonances, aligning practitioner, plant and animal energies, and spiritual intention.

On a procedural level, plant material and items relating to the animal (representative images, claws, teeth, fur, and so on) are contained together, with prayer and invocation, using shamanic skills to vitalize intention. The resonant accord among plant, animal, and practitioner is the initial focus, which is given governance and purpose through prayerful intention. If there is no real resonance there is no substantial or identifiable energy, and if there is no clear intention there is lack of reliable effect.

The list of correspondences offered here is a sampling, a springboard for your explorations. Deepening awareness of interrelationship expands spiritual practice and the realization of community. The plant names given in parenthesis are common names aiding identification.

Bat	Bat's wings (holly)
Bear	Bearberry (uva ursi)
	Bear's foot (lady's mantle)
	Bearweed (yerba santa)
	Mullein
	Leafcup
	Bear grass
Birds	Bird's eye (heart's ease)
	Bird's foot (fenugreek)
	Bird's nest (carrot)
	Celandine
	Cinquefoil

Crowberry (poke)
Daffodil
Goose grass (cleavers)
Hawkweed
Knotweed
Mallard (marshmallow)
Plantain

Goat   Goatsbeard
Goat's leaf (honeysuckle)
Goat's thorn
Goat's weed (St. Johnswort)

Cat   Catmint
Catnip
Cattail
Dandelion
Lion's foot (lady's mantle)
Lion's herb (columbine)
Pussywillow
Tiger lily
Cat's foot (ground ivy)

Deer   Corn
Deerberry (wintergreen)
Deer's tongue

Dog   Dog grass
Dog rowan tree (crampbark)
Dog rose
Dog's mercury
Dog standard (ragwort)
Dogstooth violet
Dogwood
Horehound
Hound's tongue

Dragon   Basil
Dragonsblood
Dragonwort (bistort)

	Mandragon (mandrake)
	Snapdragon
Fox	Foxglove
	Fox's clote (burdock)
	Foxtail (club moss)
Frog	Cinquefoil
Horse	Alfalfa
	Coltsfoot
	Horse chestnut
	Horse heal (elecampane)
	Horsetail
	Horse tongue
	Horse violet
Moose	Moose elm (slippery elm)
Rabbit	Gorse
	Harebell (bluebell)
	Harefoot (avens)
	Hare's ear
	Hops
	Rabbit brush
Raccoon	Coon root (bloodroot)
	Raccoon berry (may apple)
Skunk	Skunk cabbage
Snake	Adder's tongue
	Snake lily (blue flag)
	Snakeroot
	Snake's friend (Indian paintbrush)
	Snake's grass (yarrow)
Spider	Devil's club
Wolf	Wolf claw (club moss)
	Wolf's milk (euphorbia)

Herb Allies for Specific Aspects of Well-being

European herb lore is rich in its application of plant energies to a wide array of situations and issues. There is an herb for each occasion, for each need. Herbs are used as helpers in the form of amulets, or they may be advantageously placed around a room, over a doorway, or about a person. Other situations might require an herb to be burned, drunk as a beverage, applied as an ointment or wash, or stuffed into a pillow. Intention, belief, and procedure all play roles in this form of application, as does rapport with the plant or plants used.

Some herbs, such as camphor, may be used as aids for divination or burned as incense; orris root is used as a pendulum for divination; plants such as cherry, dandelion, goldenrod, ivy, and meadowsweet are associated with specific procedures used in divining particular information. Other plants, like broom, generally promote an atmosphere conducive to divinatory success.

In another category are herbs linked with courage, including borage, the flower of gladness; black cohosh; mullein; poke; thyme; tonka; and yarrow; all of which are carried and, as in the case of thyme, smelled, to help the herb's bearer be brave.

Many herbs are associated with love, an important arena in which to have allies. Herbs are used to predict, attract, enhance, and sustain love. Some potions and applications are blatantly manipulative, but love herbs can also be approached as helpers in aligning with right, joyful, fulfilling relationship, and with promotion of heart alliance in all realms. Herbs for love include alfalfa, aster, bedstraw, birch, blackberry, burdock, catnip, cherry, coltsfoot, corn, cowslip, daisy, alder, feverfew, goldenrod, iris, lady's mantle, licorice, mugwort, myrtle, oats, orris, passion flower, plantain, raspberry, rhubarb, rose, sorrel, spearmint, spikenard, strawberry, tansy, thyme, tonka, valerian, violet, and willow.

Fidelity, especially that associated with marriage, is strengthened by chickweed, clover, elder, licorice, magnolia, nutmeg, rhubarb, rye, skullcap, spikenard, and yerba maté. Another aspect of love is friendship; herbs carried or worn to attract friendship are catnip, passion flower, and sweetpea.

Catnip is considered an herb of happiness in general, as are celandine, hawthorne, lavender, marjoram, saffron, St. Johnswort, and witch grass.

Most herbs are healers of one kind or another, but, like certain people, certain herbs are particularly given to healing's priority; the presence of these herbs serves active commitment to healing. Such plants include angelica, apple, lemon balm, bay, blackberry, calamus, cedar, elder, fennel, ginseng, goldenrod, hops, horehound, mugwort, myrrh, nettle, oak, onion, plantain, peppermint, rose, rosemary, rue, sandalwood, sorrel, thistle, thyme, vervain, violet, willow, and wintergreen. Tobacco, used rightly, is also in this category.

Cypress is the tree of eternity and immortality, its medicine a blessing in both this world and the hereafter. Other herbs of longevity are lavender, maple, peach, sage, and tansy.

Carrying herbs for good luck has a long history among humans living in a unpredictable world, where it behooves one to gain allies in all realms of influence. Good luck herbs can be viewed as plants whose natures help us to find resonance with a flow attentive to well-being. These could also be thought of as herbs of synchronicity. Good luck herbs include: aloe, calamus, daffodil, fern, hazel, linden, oak, poppy, purslane, rose, oatstraw, strawberry, and violet. Chamomile is thought to give luck to gamblers.

Along with luck is the grouping of herbs linked with prosperity. These herbs in their various ways embody a truth of abundance or of the thriving that is possible in the interconnection of giving and receiving. The prosperity herbs help perspective to be open, positive, and accepting of good. Some of the plants found in the long list of prosperity herbs are alfalfa, almond, basil, cedar, chamomile, cinquefoil, clove, clover, comfrey, dill, dock, elder, fenugreek, fern, flax, ginger, goldenrod, honeysuckle, jasmine, mandrake, maple, marjoram, mint, oak, oat, Oregon grape, peas, periwinkle, pine, pipsissewa, poplar, poppy, sassafras, snakeroot, vervain, and woodruff.

Herbs known to support mental strength may, like ginko, have a direct medicinal effect on the brain, or, like eyebright, aid vision and thereby aid thought. Other herbs supportive of cognitive function in either subtle or concrete ways are caraway, celery, horehound, mustard, rosemary, rue, summer savory, spearmint, and walnut.

Various aspects of peace can be addressed using herb allies. Dulse is used to pacify sea spirits; gardenia, sprinkled in a room, promotes a peaceful atmosphere, as does lavender. Loosestrife, by its very name, speaks of the dispersal of negativity, as meadowsweet denotes the gentle power to establish peace and gladden the heart. Morning glory is another herb evocative of peace and happiness; its seeds are placed under pillows to ward off nightmares. Myrtle, grown beside the home, supports harmony within the household; olive leaves traditionally signify peace, and passion flower is used to bring calm during dispute. Pennyroyal is another herb given to remedy quarrels. Skullcap, a relaxant and anticonvulsant, brings peace to the nervous system. Vervain and valerian, also influential to the nervous system, are herbs of rest and peace, and wormwood is said to promote harmony between nations. The Greeks wore violets to calm their tempers.

In a different vein are herbs for promoting success. These are stimulating herbs like ginger or cinnamon with their warm, lively vitality and enthusiasm, or herbs like clover or lemon balm that attract good fortune. Herbs associated overall with strength are bay, mulberry, pennyroyal, plantain, St. Johnswort, and thistle.

In categories focused on spiritual or psychic strength are herbs frequently used as meditative or ceremonial incenses, such as frankincense, myrrh, sandalwood, sweetgrass, gardenia, and cinnamon; herbs that are allies of visionary experience, such as bay, damiana, kava-kava, uva ursi, wormwood, crocus, and datura; and herbs for vivid or prophetic dreaming, such as bracken, buchu, cinquefoil, heliotrope, jasmine, marigold, mimosa, mugwort, and rose. Dandelion, bay, pipsissewa, and sweetgrass are used for Spirit-calling, and angelica, violet, and coltsfoot nurture spiritual alignment. Psychic power in general is associated with bay, borage, buchu, celery, cinnamon, chicory flowers, elecampane, eyebright (those last three, along with marigold, are linked with seeing fairies), flax, honeysuckle, lemongrass, mugwort, peppermint, rose, saffron, star anise, thyme, vervain, and yarrow.

Wisdom, which hopefully accompanies or is cultivated along with psychic power, is supported by alliance with iris, peach, sage, and sunflower.

Many plants are used as purification catalysts, often in the form of bath herbs or herb washes. These include anise, bay, chamomile, hyssop, lavender, lemon, lemon verbena, parsley, rosemary, sage, thyme, valerian, and yucca. Some of those herbs are also used in the form of purifying incense, as are cedar, copal, betony, prairie sage, and tobacco. Some herbs, such as anise, hyssop, and thistle, are ingested in decoction or infusion for purifying purposes. Other plants, including bloodroot, broom, fennel, iris, mimosa, and peppermint, are carried or kept present in a room for the benefits of their purifying emanations.

A final grouping is one containing an extensive array of plants—those considered protective allies. Most of these herbs have already been listed in other categories here. Some protection herbs, such as cactus, blackberry, buckthorne, and other prickly friends, are defensive guardians. Some, like elder or datura, are uncompromisingly particular about motivation, mindfulness, and clarity. Other protection herbs, such as frankincense, lotus, and angelica, resonate with spiritual presence or, like pine and lavender, are watchful, pure, and peace-invoking. Herbs like elecampane, fern, violet, and marigold bring into play the powers of the fairy realms, and protective trees like hazel and oak are traditionally linked to Celtic magic.

All the protective herbs, whether their natures are warrior-like, deitific, diplomatic, or transformative, are allies of discernment and appropriate response. The list of these herbs includes aconite, agrimony, alfalfa, aloe, angelica, anise, bay, betony, birch, blackberry, bloodroot, blueberry, boneset, broom, buckthorne, burdock, cactus, calamus, caraway, cedar, celandine, cinquefoil, clove, cohosh, datura, dill, elder, elecampane, fennel, fern, frankincense, garlic, ginseng, hazel, heather, holly, horehound, hyssop, moss, ivy, juniper, kava-kava, lavender, linden, loosestrife, lotus, mallow, mandrake, marigold, mint, mistletoe, mugwort, mullein, mustard, myrrh, oak, orris, parsley, pennyroyal, pine, plantain, purslane, raspberry, rattlesnake root, rhubarb, rice, rose, rosemary, rue, sage, sandalwood, snapdragon, star anise, St. Johnswort, thistle, thyme, tulip, valerian, violet, wintergreen, witch hazel, wood betony, and wormwood.

Herbs Used in Ceremony

Participation in ceremony is usually preceded by purification baths. The herbs used for ceremonial cleansing are also used to wash sacred objects and to clean ritual precincts. Those herbs include: lavender, rosemary, verbena, thyme, roses, chamomile, hyssop, iris, valerian, vervain, yucca, fennel, and pine.

Smudging or censing is another ceremonial preparation involving participants, objects, and ceremonial space. Frequently called upon in this capacity are: prairie sage, cedar, myrrh, frankincense, asafoetida, sweetgrass, and copal.

During ceremony, various herbs may be burned to provide appropriate atmosphere for invocations. Those herbs, in some spiritual traditions, are grouped according to astrological affinities. During invocation of solar-related energies, sandalwood, cinnamon, saffron, cedar, copal, or frankincense may be used. Lunar incenses are: camphor, jasmine, myrrh, lily, and gardenia. Mercury herbs include narcissus, mace, and verbena; Venus incense includes cardamom, rose, and sage. For Martian invocations, pine, tobacco, or cubeb may be used; Jupiter energies resonate with agrimony, anise, and garden sage; and incenses of Saturn include datura, hemp, and patchouli. For Neptune influence, burn wild lettuce, lotus, or lobelia incense. Uranus energies are reflected in chicory, elecampane, and spikenard, while Pluto is invoked with false unicorn, ambergris, and damiana. General invocations are supported by burning worm-wood, sweetgrass, dandelion, or thistle.

Herbs are often used to companion sacred objects as part of spiritual maintenance and protection of bundles, ritual implements, or ceremonial regalia. Some of the herbs commonly used in North America for this are sweetgrass, prairie sage, lavender, rose, corn pollen, and tobacco.

To create or preserve an atmosphere of harmony and peace, certain herbs may be incorporated into ceremony as part of regalia, altar arrangements, or other elements of sacred space, or in the form of incenses/smudges, fragrant oils, or offerings. Those herbs are: gardenia, lavender, loosestrife, meadowsweet, morning glory, myrtle, olive, passion flower, pennyroyal, skull-cap, sweetgrass, vervain, violet, and rose.

A number of different herbs are employed in ceremony as visionary allies, usually in the form of smokes, incenses, salves, or teas. Those herbs include: mugwort, poplar, peyote, dittany of Crete, tobacco, cinquefoil, cedar, eyebright, chicory, rose, wormwood, angelica, damiana, kava-kava, coltsfoot, yohimbe, elecampane, datura (poisonous), henbane (poisonous); an incense blend of sandalwood, benzoin, cascarilla, vetiver, salt petre, balsam of Tolu, hemp seed, datura, psyllium seed, and violet leaves, or a mix of frankincense, myrrh, wormwood, hemp seed, St. Johnswort, coriander, anise, cardamom, mugwort, and oil of narcissus.

Traditional herbs for offering are found in many North American and European ceremonial contexts. Those herbs are most often tobacco, corn, spikenard, frankincense, myrrh, and sweetgrass.

Herbs can be used to maintain the integrity of sacred space during ceremony. The ritual precinct can be bordered by herbs, or plants can guard the directional stations. These herbs can also be burned, worn, placed on an altar, or strewn over the ritual space. Appropriate herbs for this include: angelica, basil, birch, cactus, cedar, clove, elder, fern, fleabane, garlic, spruce, sweetgrass, rosemary, horehound, juniper, mistletoe, mullein, nettle, onion, peony, pine, rue, sandalwood, thistle, and yarrow.

Ceremonial tools and structures are created from wood that is chosen for its specific spiritual as well as physical characteristics. Acacia and almond woods are generally useful; apple, ash, hazel, and rowan are frequently chosen for staffs and wands; birch is excellent for altars; elder wood is used for implements related to spirit invocation and hawthorne for implements of protection. Oak is associated with druidic ceremony. Willow is encountered in sweat lodge, hoop, and shield frames (aspen is a good shield frame also). Pine makes fine teepee lodge poles; cottonwood and cedar are used for drum bodies and frames, and cedar is used for ceremonial arbors. Spruce foliage is a traditional part of ceremonial regalia in some parts of North America.

The seasonal holy days have certain herbs associated with them that are incorporated into the ceremonial observances of those special occasions. Samhain herbs include: wormwood, cedar, bay, reeds, acorns, apple, dittany, fumitory, mullein, oak, pumpkin, and sage. Winter solstice herbs are: fir, blessed thistle, chamomile, frankincense, holly, mistletoe, pine, yew, and rosemary. On Imbolc, herbs such as angelica, basil, rowan, celandine, heather, and myrrh are used to celebrate. Herbs of the spring equinox are alder, celandine, dogwood, honeysuckle, iris, jasmine, tansy, and violet.

On Beltane use almond, frankincense, ivy, marigold, meadowsweet, rose, woodruff, and willow. Herbs for summer solstice include chamomile, elder, fennel, lavender, mugwort, St. Johnswort, verbena, wormwood, vervain, oak, and heather. Lughnasad is celebrated with fenugreek, corn, frankincense, heather, hollyhock, oak, and sunflower. The autumn equinox resonates with benzoin, fern, milkweed, myrrh, passion flower, sage, Solomon's seal, thistle, squash, gourds, wheat, aspen, corn, and apples.

Suggested Reading

The herbs discussed in this text were chosen for their common usage. Consult local resources in your exploration of the plants that grow in your bioregion. Ethnobotany texts can be found in local museums or through native plant societies. Indigenous knowledge is invaluable to the shamanic herbalist.

Texts can be very helpful to the herbalist. Here are a few points to consider when taking on a text (that is, an author) as your teacher or consultant.

Some texts are original works but most are rearrangements of existing information copied from other books. As you gain experience in reading herbal texts, it becomes obvious whether the information was gained from experience or derived from other books. Some experiential knowledge is too idiosyncratic, or perhaps too biased by preconditioning, to be of general use to others, though aspects may be inspiring or provocative. Studying the work of other practitioners yields insights, may add to your repertoire of remedies, and broadens your healing perspective. It also furthers the sense and the reality of the healing community. Texts that are mainly compilations of information derived from other books are most helpful for novice herbalists and for those having extensive practical experience and knowledge. These texts vary widely in quality and technical level, and most are based on the naturopathic perspective.

The author's background and the historical context in which a book is written influence, to various degrees, the attitudes and information presented. Be aware of subtle opinions put forth by the author. Get a feel for her relationship to plants, her approach to health, her fears and prejudices, where her knowledge has come from, and who she perceives her readers to be. Those factors color the knowledge presented in the text.

To be useful, a good herbal text should list Latin as well as common names, and include a comprehensive index. Specialist authors are often the best resource for specialized information, such as information on herbs for childbirth, food herbs, dye herbs, and so on. Those authors usually write from considerable experience and interest in their fields.
Specific information about doses, preparation, and application make a big difference in how useful a book is to the practicing herbalist. Some books focus on ailments, some on formulas. When using your resources, use each for its strength—do not expect to find one perfect text. The more familiar you become with your texts, the easier it is to know which one to turn to for certain types of information. Each has its good points and its shortcomings. The authors of your oft-used texts become like friends whose voices are familiar and whose fine qualities you know.

Recognize how your local plant environment relates to the bioregion the author is surrounded by. Remember, each time you use an herb you are learning, and this experiential knowledge is valid. Sometimes information from the past no longer applies, or applies in different ways as your life, and the world, change.

James Adams. *Landscaping with Herbs.* Portland, Or.: Timber Press, 1987.

Jeannine Parvati Baker. *Hygeia: A Woman's Herbal.* San Francisco: Wildwood House, 1978.

Dan Bensky and Andrew Gamble. *Chinese Herbal Medicine: Materia Medica.* Seattle: Eastland Press, 1993.

Philip M. Chancellor. *Dr. Phillip M. Chancellor's Handbook of the Bach Flower Remedies.* New Canaan, Conn.: Keats, 1980.

John R. Christopher. *School of Natural Healing.* Provo, Ut.: BiWorld, 1976.

Juliette de Bairacli Levy. *Common Herbs for Natural Health.* Woodstock, N.Y.: Ash Tree, 1996.

Harvey Wickes Felter and John Lloyd Jr. *King's American Dispensatory,* 18th edition, vol. 1 and 2. Portland: Eclectic Medical Publications, 1983.

Steven Foster. *Herbal Bounty! The Gentle Art of Herb Culture.* Salt Lake City: G.M. Smith, 1984.

Frater Albertus. *The Alchemist's Handbook: Manual for Practical Laboratory Alchemy.* York Beach, Me.: Samuel Weiser, 1974.

Ingrid Gabriel. *Herb Identifier and Handbook.* New York: Sterling, 1975.

Maude Grieve. *A Modern Herbal.* New York: Dover, 1978.

Paul Hawken. *The Magic of Findhorn.* London: Souvenir, 1975.

Jean Hersey. *The Woman's Day Book of Wildflowers.* New York: Simon and Schuster, 1976.

David Hoffman. *The Complete Illustrated Holistic Herbal: A Safe and Practical Guide to Making and Using Herbal Remedies.* Rockport, Mass.: Element Books, 1996.

Alma R. Hutchens. *Indian Herbalogy of North America.* Boston: Shambhala, 1991.

Manfred M. Junius. *The Practical Handbook of Plant Alchemy: An Herbalist's Guide to Preparing Medicinal Essences, Tinctures, and Elixirs.* Rochester, Vt.: Healing Arts Press, 1993.

Vasant Lad. *The Yoga of Herbs: An Ayurvedic Guide to Herbal Medicine.* Sante Fe: Lotus, 1986.

John B. Lust. *The Herb Book.* New York: B. Lust, 1974.

Charles Frederick Millspaugh. *American Medicinal Plants: An Illustrated and Descriptive Guide to Plants Indigenous to and Naturalized in the United States Which Are Used in Medicine.* New York: Dover, 1974.

David Moerman. *Medicinal Plants of Native America.* University of Michigan Museum of Anthropology, technical reports, number 19. Ann Arbor Mi., 1986

James Mooney. *The Swimmer Manuscript of Cherokee Sacred Formulas and Medicinal Prescriptions.* Capilola, Calif.: Botanical Press.

Michael Moore. *Medicinal Plants of the Mountain West: A Guide to the Identification, Preparation, and Uses of Traditional Medicinal Plants Found in the Mountains, Foothills, and Upland Areas of the American West.* Santa Fe: Museum of New Mexico Press, 1979.

Gary Paul Nabhan. *Enduring Seeds: Native American Agriculture and Wild Plant Conservation.* San Francisco: North Point Press, 1989.

Henrietta A. Diers Rau. *Healing with Herbs: Nature's Way to Better Health.* New York: Arco, 1976.

Richard Evans Schultes. *Medicines from the Earth: A Guide to Healing Plants.* New York: Alfred van der Marck, 1983.

Michael Tierra. *Planetary Herbology: An Integration of Western Herbs into the Traditional Chinese and Ayurvedic Systems.* Twin Lakes Wi.: Lotus, 1988.

Virgil J. Vogel. *American Indian Medicine.* Norman: University of Oklahoma Press, 1970.

Susun S. Weed. *Wise Woman Herbal: Healing Wise.* Woodstock, N.Y.: Ash Tree, 1989.

Terry Willard. *Edible and Medicinal Plants of the Rockies and Neighboring Territories.* Calgary, Alberta: Wild Rose College of Natural Healing, 1992.

Gilbert Wilson. *Buffalo Woman's Garden.* St. Paul: Minnesota Historical Society, 1987.

Sources of Supply

Sources for Seeds & Plants

Abundant Life Seed Foundation
P.O. Box 772, Port Townsend WA 98368
360-385-5660
Specializing in open-pollinated, organic heirloom seeds of herbs, vegetables, flowers, grains, wildflowers, trees, and shrubs. A nonprofit foundation dedicated to the preservation of genetic diversity.

Bountiful Gardens
18001 Shafer Ranch Road, Willits CA 95490-9626
707-459-6410
Specializing in untreated and open-pollinated seeds, heirloom varieties. Biointensive and organic gardening publications and supplies.

Companion Plants
7247 N. Coolville Ridge, Athens OH 45701
614-592-4643
Over six hundred varieties of herbs. Send $3.00 for catalog.

Fedco Seeds
P.O. Box 520, Waterville ME 04903
A consumer/worker-owned co-op specializing in untreated seeds for short growing seasons and cold climates. Root stock available for medicinal plants. Send $2.00 for catalog.

Meadowbrook Herb Garden
93 Kingstown Road, Wyoming RI 02898
401-539-7603
Certified biodynamic and organic growers of culinary herbs.

Native Seeds/Search
2509 N. Campbell Avenue #325, Tuscon AZ 85719
520-327-9123
Specializing in heirloom crops of the greater Southwest. Send
$1.00 for catalog. Also prints *Seedhead News,* a good source for
Southwest and American Indian herb information.

Nichols Garden Nursery
1190 N. Pacific Highway, Albany OR 97301
541-928-9280
Specializing in herbs and rare seeds for home gardeners.

Redwood City Seed Company
P.O. Box 361, Redwood City CA 94064
415-325-7333
Specializing in endangered cultivated plants, especially heirloom vegetables and unusual culinary and medicinal herbs.

Sandy Mush Herb Nursery
316 Surrett Cove Road, Leicester NC 28748-5517
704-683-2014
Specializing in herbs, native plants, and perennials. Send $5.00
for catalog.

Fresh & Dried Herbs & Herbal Remedies

All these businesses have catalogs available; I suggest you en-
close $1.00 with requests—many of these listings are for small
family-operated businesses.

Blessed Herbs
109 Barre Plains Road, Oakham MA 01068
508-882-3839 / 800-489-4372
Wholesale organic and wildcrafted herbs and extracts. Selection and quality are excellent.

Equinox Botanicals
333446 McCumber Road, Rutland OH 45775
614-742-2548
Carefully made medicinal tinctures, teas, and salves from organic and wildcrafted herbs.

Fairewood Botanicals
P.O. Box 1273, Freeland WA 98249
360-579-8963
Hand-harvested fresh-plant extracts and oils from native herbs of the Northwest. Large selection of quality wild and organic dried herbs.

Frontier Coop Herbs
Box 299, Norway IA 52318
800-669-3275
Large selection of wholesale herbs and related products.

Green Terrestrial
P.O. Box 266, Milton NY 12547
914-795-5238
Botanicals from the wise woman tradition. Apprenticeship program offered.

Herb Pharm
P.O. Box 116, Williams OR 97544
541-846-6262
Organic medicinal plants, herbal extracts, and herbal health care products.

Loren Cruden
P.O. Box 218, Orient WA 99160
Correspondence by mail only.
Workshops, books, Living Earth Tarot.

Mountain Spirit
P.O. Box 368, Port Townsend WA 98368
360-385-4491 / 800-817-7233
Organic and wildcrafted herbs, remedies, and related items. Specializing in herbal remedies for women and children. Good selection, service, and prices.

Red Moon Herbs
P.O. Box 780, Leicester NC 28748
Correspondence by mail only.
Medicinal vinegars, extracts, oils, and salves made from wildcrafted and organically cultivated plants, prepared by hand in the wise woman tradition. Select dried herbs also available. Personal service.

Ryan Drum
Waldron Island, WA 98297
Correspondence by mail only.
Teacher and wildcrafter; fine quality herbs.

Wild Botanicals
P.O. Box 2264, Corvallis OR 97339
541-929-4753
Good selection of organic and wildcrafted dried herbs and seeds. Agroforestry consulting, sustainable harvesting.

Plant Index

General Index